Health
Matters

for People with Developmental Disabilities

Health Matters

for People with Developmental Disabilities

Creating a Sustainable Health Promotion Program

by

Beth Marks, RN, Ph.D.

Jasmina Sisirak, M.P.H

and

Tamar Heller, Ph.D.
Rehabilitation Research and Training Center on Aging
with Developmental Disabilities
Department of Disability and Human Development
University of Illinois at Chicago

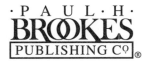

·P·A·U·L·H·
BROOKES
PUBLISHING CO ®

Baltimore • London • Sydney

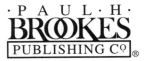

Paul H. Brookes Publishing Co.
Post Office Box 10624
Baltimore, Maryland 21285-0624
USA

www.brookespublishing.com

Typeset by Spearhead Global, Inc., Bear, Delaware.
Manufactured in the United States of America by
Sheridan Books, Inc., Chelsea, Michigan.

Funded by U.S. Department of Education, Office of Special Education and Rehabilitative Services,
National Institute on Disability and Rehabilitation Research, Grants H133B980046 and H133B031134;
Centers for Disease Control and Prevention's Disability and Health Branch, Grant C CRS514155;
National Institute on Aging, Grants P50 AG15890-12 and P30 AG22849-01; and the Retirement
Research Foundation, Grant 2003-119. The contents of this book do not necessarily represent the
policy of the U.S. Department of Education and should not be viewed as an endorsement by the
Federal government.

Library of Congress Cataloging-in-Publication Data

Marks, Beth.
  Health matters for people with developmental disabilities : creating a sustainable health promotion
program / by Beth Marks, Jasmina Sisirak, and Tamar Heller.
     p.   cm.
  Includes bibliographical references and index.
  ISBN-13: 978-1-59857-000-7 (pbk.)
  ISBN-10: 1-59857-000-5 (pbk.)
  1. Developmentally disabled—Health and hygiene—United States.   2. Health promotion—United
States.   I. Sisirak, Jasmina.   II. Heller, Tamar.   III. Title.
  [DNLM: 1. Developmental Disabilities—United States.   2. Health Promotion—organization &
administration—United States.   3. Health Planning—methods—United States.   4. Health Status
Disparities—United States.   5. Organizational Innovation—United States.   6. Program Evaluation—
standards—United States. WA 525 M346h 2010]
  HV3006.A4M265 2010
  362.196'8—dc22   2010009136

British Library Cataloguing in Publication data are available from the British Library.

2014   2013   2012   2011   2010

10   9   8   7   6   5   4   3   2   1

Contents

About the Authors

Beth Marks, RN, Ph.D., Research Assistant Professor, Department of Disability and Human Development, University of Illinois at Chicago, 1640 West Roosevelt Road, Chicago, Illinois, 60608

Dr. Marks is also Associate Director for Research in the Rehabilitation Research and Training Center on Aging with Developmental Disabilities (RRTCADD) and President of the National Organization of Nurses with Disabilities. She directs research activities related to health promotion, health advocacy, primary health care, and occupational health and safety for persons with intellectual and developmental disabilities. Dr. Marks has developed and implemented community-based surveys related to health and safety for people with disabilities and has written publications and presented papers in the area of disability, health, and community engagement in the United States and internationally. She has coedited a special issue for *Nursing Clinics of North America* titled *Promoting Health Across the Lifespan for Persons with Developmental Disabilities* and a feasibility study report, *Advancing Nursing Education at Bel-Air Sanatorium and Hospital in Panchgani, Maharashtra, India*, through The Global Health Leadership Office/ WHO Collaborating Center at the University of Illinois at Chicago.

Jasmina Sisirak, M.P.H., Associate Project Director, Department of Disability and Human Development, University of Illinois at Chicago, 1640 West Roosevelt Road, Chicago, Illinois, 60608

Ms. Sisirak's research interests focus on nutrition, health literacy, and health promotion for persons with intellectual and developmental disabilities. She coordinates several health promotion projects in the Rehabilitation Research and Training Center on Aging with Developmental Disabilities and has written publications and has presented papers in the area of disability in the DHD at UIC. Her research interests consist of nutrition, health literacy, and health promotion for persons with intellectual and developmental disabilities. She coordinates several health promotion projects in the RRTCADD and has written publications and presented papers in the areas of disability, health, and nutrition. Ms. Sisirak received her bachelor of science degree in dietetics at Southern Illinois University and her master of public health at UIC. Currently, she is a doctoral candidate in community health sciences in the School of Public Health at the University of Illinois at Chicago.

Tamar Heller, Ph.D., Professor and Head, Department of Disability and Human Development, University of Illinois at Chicago, and Director of the Institute on Disability and Human Development, the University Center of Excellence in Developmental Disabilities, 1640 West Roosevelt Road, Chicago, Illinois, 60608

Dr. Heller also directs the Rehabilitation Research and Training Center on Aging with Developmental Disabilities and projects on support interventions for individuals with disabilities, including the Special Olympics Research Collaborating Center. Dr. Heller has written more than 150 publications and presented more than 200 papers at major conferences on family support interventions and policies, self-determination, health promotion, and aging of people with developmental disabilities. She has coedited two books (*Health of Women with Intellectual Disabilities*, Blackwell Publishing, 2002; *Older Adults with Developmental Disabilities: Optimizing Choice and Change*, Paul H. Brookes Publishing Co., 1993) and edited special issues of *Technology and Disability, American Journal on Mental Retardation, Journal of Policy and Practice in Intellectual Disabilities*, and *Family Relations*. She is the president of the board of the Association of University Centers on Disabilities. In 2005 she was a delegate to the White House Conference on Aging. As a cofounder of the national Sibling Leadership Network, she is a member of its steering committee. Her awards include the 2009 Autism Ally for Public Policy Award of The Arc/The Autism Program of Illinois; the 2008 Lifetime Research Achievement Award, International Association for the Scientific Study of Intellectual Disabilities, Special Interest Group on Aging and Intellectual Disabilities; and the 2009 Community Partner Award of Community Support Services.

Foreword

People with developmental disabilities (DD) will more fully participate in their communities when they are not constrained by poor health and they can access the necessary resources and power to change conditions affecting their health status. A fundamental question is whether we believe that people with DD have the right to attain the highest standard of health or whether we accept the inequities in health care and health status experienced by the vast majority of people with DD worldwide. On a global level, the United Nations (UN) Convention on the Rights of Persons with Disabilities supports the impetus for *Health Matters for People with Developmental Disabilities: Creating a Sustainable Health Promotion Program* with its 50 articles addressing the human rights and fundamental freedoms that must be guaranteed for all people with disabilities to enjoy the highest attainable standard of health without discrimination. Specifically, Article 25 in the UN Convention addresses health issues and the need to take all appropriate measures to ensure access for people with disabilities to health services that are gender-sensitive, including health-related rehabilitation. *Health Matters for People with Developmental Disabilities* recognizes the importance of culturally appropriate health services, health education, and health-related information as a means of reducing disparities in health status for people with DD.

Although the deinstitutionalization movement supported individuals with disabilities to live in community settings with rights and opportunities for education, recreation, employment, and housing, the social and environmental supports needed for healthy lifestyles were not often considered. Consequently, people with DD continue to have widening inequities in health care services compared with their peers without disabilities, as well as poorer health outcomes. Despite the documented benefit of health promotion and education to maintain health and control risk factors, people with DD continue to be excluded from many community-based health promotion programs.

In 2002, the Surgeon General held a conference on Health Disparities and Mental Retardation to identify strategies to improve health status among people with DD across the lifespan and issued several goals to improve access to health care services in their communities. Two key goals aimed to 1) integrate health promotion into community environments of people with DD and 2) increase knowledge and understanding of health through practical and useful information. As such, people with DD need innovative strategies and solutions to address priority areas and challenge the many barriers they face in obtaining appropriate health care services. These barriers range from exclusion in public campaigns promoting wellness, shortages of health care professionals who are willing to accept them as patients and understand their unique needs, and access barriers (e.g., programmatic, attitudinal, physical, and communication barriers). From an ecological perspective this means care that focuses on individuals, families, communities, and organizational/cultural and policy components of a health care system that facilitate care and optimal health. The authors of this text are a multidisciplinary team committed to using the best evidence available, along with their considerable expertise in caring for underserved and underrepresented people, to deliver a work that helps us think in theoretical and practical ways that will optimize the health of people with DD.

This book provides easy-to-use and accessible information on the topics related to health, including the areas essential for building a tailored health promotion program empowering individuals to express their health concerns, which is critical in gaining control over one's health. In addition, the challenges in developing and implementing health promotion programs are discussed, along with strategies that can be used by community-based service providers to implement programs. For people with DD, health information is needed to reduce their fears and to support them in making informed health care choices. A particular strength of *Health Matters for People with Developmental Disabilities* is the attention to a health system that epitomizes Primary Health Care (PHC) as that term is defined by the World Health Organization (WHO) and others. In other words, it advocates a health care system that ensures essential care for all that is culturally acceptable and appropriate, accessible, affordable, and that engages the active participation of community members. The information in this book included input from people with DD and their support people in community settings. A primary emphasis is placed on accessibility and affordability. Much of the information provided in this text incorporates materials that can be found in any household.

It is important to view health as a fundamental right for all. The authors of *Health Matters for People with Developmental Disabilities* help us achieve these global goals at a local level of implementation by providing a step-by-step resource manual for creating sustainable health promotion programs. Within that perspective, the design of services must ensure dignity and enhance the capacity of people with DD to make informed choices for ensuring optimal health. Implementing successful health promotion programs requires consideration of factors that support or inhibit people with DD from initiating and maintaining healthy behaviors. Because personal health practices are just one of the determinants of health, programs must address environmental, cultural, and psychosocial constraints that affect individuals and their support people. Integrating health promotion strategies within existing community-based structures, such as schools, churches, worksite settings, day programs, and residential programs for people with DD can provide the structure for continuous access to information, ongoing financial support, and participation in health promoting behaviors.

Beverly J. McElmurry, Ed.D., FAAN
Professor and Associate Dean
Director, WHO Collaborating Centre for
International Nursing Development in Primary Health Care

Preface

Health Matters for People with Developmental Disabilities: Creating a Sustainable Health Promotion Program is based on the successful outcomes of the innovative 5-year (2003–2008) University of Illinois at Chicago (UIC) Train-the-Trainer Health Promotion research program for staff in community-based organizations to enhance health status, increase physical activity, and improve food choices in settings in which people with DD work and live. The goals of the program were to 1) start and implement a 12-week physical activity and health education program using *Health Matters: The Exercise and Nutrition Health Education Curriculum for People with Developmental Disabilities* (Marks et al., 2010), 2) learn how to motivate and engage adults with developmental disabilities (DD)* in a physical activity and health education program, 3) teach core concepts of physical activity and nutrition to adults with DD, and 4) support adults with DD to incorporate physical activity and healthy lifestyles into activities of daily living. Staff in community-based organizations received an 8-hour, small-group (7–10 staff), on-site Health Matters Train-the-Trainer Workshop. The training was given to staff immediately before they started the 12-week health promotion program for adults with DD. Technical assistance from the UIC research team was provided to staff throughout the duration of the 12-week program via phone, e-mail, and site visits.

The principal investigator for this study was Beth Marks. Tamar Heller was coinvestigator and Jasmina Sisirak served as Project Coordinator. This project demonstrated the capacity of staff to change health-related behaviors and improve the health status of their clients with DD and of themselves (Marks et al., 2008; Marks et al., 2007). Ninety-one participants with DD and 66 staff from six different community-based organizations in Illinois and New Mexico participated in the study. The intervention group included 51 participants with DD and 41 staff, and the control group included 40 people with DD and 25 staff. Results showed significant changes in psychosocial health status, including decreased perceived pain, increased self-efficacy and social/environmental supports, improved cholesterol and fasting glucose levels, improved flexibility, and improvements in waist-to-hip ratio. After the program, staff participants had significantly higher outcome expectations of exercise and nutrition for themselves. In addition, staff had significantly more support for nutrition following the program and a higher intake of fruits and vegetables.

---

*For the purpose of this book, we primarily use the term *developmental disabilities* (DD) to encompass both developmental disabilities and intellectual disabilities (ID).

Aims of the Book

Health Matters for People with Developmental Disabilities: Creating a Sustainable Health Promotion Program is a compilation of over a decade of lessons learned that will help you and your organization establish a community-based health promotion program for adults with DD. As service providers, administrators, researchers, policy makers, and government officials embrace the power of health promotion activities in transforming lives among people with disabilities, structured approaches are needed in order to implement sustainable health promotion programs. Implementation of health promotion activities is critical to the success of efforts to integrate and maintain people with DD in community settings. Adults with DD will achieve community engagement more fully when they are not constrained by poor health and can command the necessary power to change conditions affecting their health status (Kalnins, McQueen, Backett, Curtice, & Currie, 1992).

Improved health education, health literacy, and appropriate environmental supports are critical components for people with DD to gain control over their health and health determinants, manage chronic conditions, and advocate for their rights as full citizens within their communities (World Health Organization, 2001). Education combined with opportunities for lifelong learning can help people with DD develop the skills and confidence they need to adapt and maintain healthy lifestyles as they age. In addition, education for caregivers about health-related issues is especially salient for individuals with DD to achieve higher health status levels (Heller & Marks, 2002). As noted by the WHO *Global Strategy for Health for All by the Year 2000* (World Health Organization, 1999) supporting these efforts, health science and technology have reached a point in which their contributions to further improve health standards can only make a real impact if people themselves become full partners in health protection and promotion.

Health Matters for People with Developmental Disabilities is a guide for promoting the health and improving health outcomes of people with DD, employees, and community-based organizations. This book presents an overview of the health status and health care disparities that exist for people with disabilities to assist readers in understanding the role that health promotion has in improving the health outcomes of these individuals and controlling the social and financial costs associated with inaccessible and unacceptable health care services. *Health Matters for People with Developmental Disabilities* combines the theoretical components related to health promotion with many practical applications and user friendly tools to delineate a step-by-step approach to planning, implementing, and evaluating your health promotion program within your organization.

Specifically, this book aims to give staff in community-based organizations the skills, knowledge, and abilities to 1) develop, organize, and implement a tailored physical activity and health education program for adults with DD; 2) evaluate the capacity of your organization and employees to do health promotion activities; 3) develop a strategic plan for health promotion in your organization to support people with DD to achieve and maintain healthy lifestyles long-term through a sustainable program; 4) implement a health promotion program for people with DD; and 5) identify and connect with community resources and funding sources to keep your health promotion program going.

We provide structured information for people to do the following activities:

1. Review key concepts related to teaching and monitoring physical activity and nutrition for adults with DD (e.g., heart rate, blood pressure, use of equipment, safety).

2. Identify and monitor the relationship of behavior change and organizational culture (e.g., staff knowledge, attitudes, beliefs) and individual health status and behaviors.

3. Set realistic goals for your organization and participants with DD.

4. Design and tailor an individualized health promotion program to encourage participants with DD to make lifestyle changes (e.g., increase physical activity, make healthy food choices).

5. Encourage and support participants to make and maintain long-term lifestyle changes (e.g., increase physical activity, make healthy food choices).

Audience

Readers of this book should have an interest in developing sustainable health promotion programs tailored to the unique needs of people with disabilities. For these individuals, health promotion has the same potential to improve physical, mental, and social functioning and to prevent the onset of lifestyle-related conditions as it does in the general population. Readers should also have an interest in understanding how the current system of care and support for people with DD is heavily influenced by existing negative and outmoded attitudes toward aging and disability, limited social supports, lack of understanding regarding unique needs, and difficulty accessing appropriate services. Each reader should have an interest in understanding the pivotal role that management in community-based day/residential support programs and direct support workers have in providing the necessary supports to obtain and maintain personal skills and behavioral choices that affect health status. Last, readers should have an interest in understanding that with support, people with disabilities—similar to their peers without disabilities—can contribute to their own well-being by becoming knowledgeable about their health and health care resources and being active participants in health promotion activities that are based on their individual needs and lifestyle preferences.

Organization

Today, improving outcomes of health care services for people with DD requires a process of *moving what we have learned* through research to *applying that knowledge* in a variety of practice settings that serve individuals with DD (Sudsawad, 2007). Creation of new knowledge during research often does not result in the implementation and sustainability of new ways of practice in the community. Knowledge Translation (KT) is a critical component of changing practice and driving improvements in health status. By using theories and conceptual frameworks to guide the translation of research results to practice settings, we provide you with a map that will aid you in planning and implementing tailored programs, evaluating the reasons for successes (or failures), and improving the programs.

The chapters in this book are structured to correspond to the stages outlined in the Transtheoretical Model of Behavior Change (Prochaska & DiClemente, 1992; Prochaska, DiClemente, & Norcross, 1992) so that the reader can learn the practical processes of the Transtheoretical Model in modifying or changing health behaviors on an individual as well as an organizational level. The Transtheoretical approach to behavior change uses five stages in which one becomes increasingly more motivated and ready to modify or change a particular behavior. The five stages consist of 1) Precontemplation, 2) Contemplation, 3) Preparation, 4) Action, and 5) Maintenance.

In the Precontemplation Stage, people are often unaware or underaware of the need to change their behavior. Chapter 1 gives an overview of important issues related to physical activity and healthy food choices that provide an impetus for starting a health promotion program for adults with DD. As people move into the Contemplation Stage, they become increasingly aware that they should change their behavior, and they are starting to assess the impact of their behavior(s). Although people are thinking about change, they have not yet made a commitment to take action.

Chapter 2 incorporates the theme of assessment by reviewing the relationship of the health status and behaviors, staff knowledge, attitudes, and beliefs (e.g., pros and cons of physical activity and healthy foods), and organizational culture of people with DD on their behavior change and healthy lifestyles.

As people gain a greater appreciation of the pros and cons related to specific behaviors, people are more inclined to take action. Behavior change will be more successful if they make plans to change a specific behavior and develop goals. This is known as the Preparation Stage. In Chapter 3, we begin to identify strategies that can be used to set realistic goals within your organization that will support individuals with DD to develop their own goals aimed at changing or modifying their health behaviors related to engaging in physical activity and making healthy food choices.

Chapter 4 corresponds to the Action Stage, in which people are taking action; have changed their behavior(s); and are looking at ways to support their new behaviors, such as exercising and trying to include healthy foods in their diets. This chapter will provide the steps to design a program that is tailored to organizational needs to encourage individuals with DD to become more physically active and to make healthy food choices.

The last chapter, Chapter 5, integrates the fifth stage, the Maintenance Stage. We discuss practical strategies for keeping your health promotion program for individuals with DD going and for supporting people in considering ways to maintain healthy behaviors and new lifestyles.

The principles of Bandura's Social Cognitive Theory are also integrated throughout all of the chapters. With Social Cognitive Theory, readers can gain insight into how movement toward behavior change is affected by one's 1) perception of the pros and cons of change, 2) confidence in the ability to change, and 3) perceived level of social support to adopt a new behavior (Bandura, 1986, 1997). Although the stages of behavior change are presented in a linear fashion within the book, the processes of behavior change are dynamic in that people often move in and out of stages that are often dependent on life events.

Learning Tools

Each chapter includes a discussion on the use of a variety of tools and measures that have been developed over the past decade through several research and training projects conducted by staff in the Rehabilitation and Research Training Center on Aging and Developmental Disabilities. For example, tools include sample timelines and budgets, staffing/personnel grids, the Organizational and Employee Capacity Checklist, and curricular materials that can be used to support your health promotion initiative.

We also developed this book for use in tandem with *Health Matters: The Exercise, Nutrition, and Health Education Curriculum for People with Developmental Disabilities*. That curriculum has 37 interactive lessons in five units—each on a different topic—that can be implemented over a 12-week period for individuals with DD. Each lesson builds on the previous one, which allows participants to continually review material throughout the program. The curriculum is designed so that the instructor can duplicate and distribute worksheets and handouts and includes a CD-ROM with all of these materials and more.

The *Health Matters* curriculum is based on the successful outcomes of the innovative University of Illinois at Chicago (UIC) 12-week *Health Promotion Program for Adults with Developmental Disabilities* that was developed and tested at the UIC from 1998 through 2003. This evidence-based program includes exercise, health education, and nutrition components. The program goals included the following: 1) improve fitness; 2) increase knowledge about healthy lifestyles; and 3) teach staff, family, and friends how to support participants to achieve these goals. Participants participated in a comprehensive program consisting of exercise and health education classes, peer support, and nutrition classes. It was tested on 62 participants from six different vocational and residential agencies in Illinois (Heller, Hsieh, & Rimmer, 2004; Rimmer, Heller, Wang, & Valerio, 2004). Results have demonstrated the following changes for participants: improved cardiovascular fitness, increased muscle strength and endurance, greater life satisfaction and less depression, more positive attitudes toward exercise, increased confidence in ability to exercise, and fewer cognitive-emotional barriers preventing participants from exercising.

References

Bandura, A. (1986). *Social foundations of thought and action: A social cognitive theory.* Upper Saddle River, NJ: Prentice Hall.

Bandura, A. (1997). Editorial: The anatomy of stages of changes. *American Journal of Health Promotion, 12,* 8–10.

Heller, T., Hsieh, K., & Rimmer, J.H. (2004). Attitudinal and psychological outcomes of a fitness and health education program on adults with Down syndrome. *American Journal on Mental Retardation, 109*(2), 175–185.

Heller, T., & Marks, B., (2002). Health promotion and women. In P.N. Walsh & T. Heller (Eds.), *Health promotion and women with intellectual disabilities* (pp. 170–189). London: Blackwell Science Publishing.

Kalnins, I., McQueen, D.V., Backett, K.C., Curtice, L., & Currie, C.E. (1992). Children, empowerment, and health promotion: Some new directions in research and practice. *Health Promotion International, 7,* 53–59.

Marks, B., Sisirak, J., & Heller, T. (2008, August). *Efficacy of a Train-the-Trainer Program on caregivers' health status, perceptions, and behavior.* Paper presented the IASSID 13th World Congress, People with Intellectual Disabilities: Citizens of the World, Cape Town, South Africa.

Marks, B., Sisirak, J., & Heller, T. (2010). *Health matters: The exercise and nutrition health education curriculum for people with developmental disabilities.* Baltimore: Paul H. Brookes Publishing Co.

Marks, B., Sisirak, J., Heller, T., & Riley, B. (2007, November). *Impact of a train-the-trainer program on the psychosocial health status of staff supporting adults with intellectual and developmental disabilities.* Paper presented at the meeting of the American Public Health Association, 135th Annual Meeting and Exposition, Washington, DC.

Melville, C.A., Cooper, S.A., McGrother, C.W., Thorp, C.F., & Collacott, R. (2005). Obesity in adults with Down syndrome: A case–control study. *Journal of Intellectual Disability Research, 49*(2), 125–133.

Prochaska, J.O., & DiClemente, C.C. (1992). Stages of change in the modification of problem behaviors. *Progress in Behavior Modification, 28,* 183–218.

Prochaska, J.O., DiClemente, C.C., & Norcross, J.C. (1992). In search of how people change: Applications to addictive behavior. *American Psychologist, 47,* 1102–1114.

Rimmer, J.H., Heller, T., Wang, E., & Valerio, I. (2004). Improvements in physical fitness in adults with Down syndrome. *American Journal of Mental Retardation, 109*(2), 165–174.

Sudsawad, P. (2007). *Knowledge translation: Introduction to models, strategies, and measures.* Austin, TX: Southwest Educational Development Laboratory, National Center for the Dissemination of Disability Research.

World Health Organization. (1999). *Health 21—Health for All in the 21st Century.* Copenhagen: World Health Organization.

World Health Organization. (2001). *Health promotion: Report by the Secretariat.* Paper presented at the 54th World Health Assembly, Geneva, Switzerland.

Acknowledgments

We would like to acknowledge the work of several people in the community for their ongoing commitment aimed at ensuring sustainability of health promotion for people with developmental disabilities to achieve improved health status and community participation: Kathrine Brinkmeier, Jeanne Desjardins, Dina Donohue-Chase, Leslie Hoelzel, Edward Kaul, and Meg Maurer. In addition, we acknowledge the work conducted by the dedicated program staff of the University of Illinois at Chicago Health Matters Program. The Health Matters Train-the-Trainer Program was developed and instructed by Beth Marks and Jasmina Sisirak. Karen Batty, Tanya Melich-Munyan and Terri Plachy provided their nursing expertise. Yen-Ching Chang, Barbara Cole, Erika Mercantonio, Yesenia Perez, and Orlando Torres provided assistance in day-to-day project operations.

*To people with intellectual and developmental
disabilities and their support staff in community-based organizations.
Our gratitude is extended to all of the people who participated in the
research projects that formed the foundation for developing the
information and resources in this text.
Without their participation and feedback, this
work would have never been possible.*

Health Promotion and Health Status

Promoting health is a key element for bridging equity gaps and advocating for policies supporting adults with developmental disabilities (DD) to achieve optimal health and wellness (Pan American Health Organization, 2001). Although health is a basic component of human development, health promotion involves a broader scope of action than that customarily handled by health care services and is essential in addressing individual and community health concerns (Pan American Health Organization, 2002). *Health promotion* is the process of enabling people to take control over and to improve their health (World Health Organization, 2002).

> Health promotion is the process of enabling people to take control over and to improve their health.

This chapter provides an overview of factors contributing to health and wellness for individuals with DD in the United States and discusses the importance of developing a comprehensive health promotion program that includes health education, nutrition, and exercise to improve the lives of adults with DD. In addition, factors related to physical activity, fitness, nutrition, and diets for individuals with DD are presented.

Supporting Rights and Health Advocacy for Adults with Developmental Disabilities

People with disabilities and their families have fought for their rights in all areas of community life, including education, employment, housing, recreation, and commerce. Although access to health care services, health promotion, and disease prevention activities is key to being able to achieve successful community engagement, people with disabilities often struggle to obtain health care services that are accessible (e.g., affordable, available) and acceptable (e.g., culturally relevant, satisfactory). In addition, many health disparities exist for people with DD due to underdiagnosis, misdiagnosis, likelihood of receiving prompt treatment, limited access to providers, lack of research information, transportation barriers, and inaccessible medical equipment (U.S. Department of Health and Human Services, 2001).

With the critical need for equality in health care services for people with DD, agencies supporting individuals with disabilities may assume a leadership role within their communities to advocate for improved access to quality health care services, such as primary care, health promotion, and disease prevention. Service providers can play a role in meeting the many training needs related to improving health literacy among people with DD and their families/support people. Community providers may also collaborate with academic institutions to meet the educational needs of professional caregivers and health care providers.

Defining Health from a Disability Perspective

People have many ideas about the meaning of *health*. Although health and social service professionals often define health for people with disabilities using a unidimensional domain—the absence of disease or impairment—individuals with DD have multidimensional views of health (Marks, 1996; Marks, Sisirak, & Hsieh, 2008), as do people in the general population. Professionals are trained to define health for people with disabilities based on etiology, diagnosis, physical changes, and treatment, which differ from people in the general population whose definitions include influences from daily life (Hornsten, Sandstrom, & Lundman, 2004). Understanding how people define their own health is critical because it can result in conflicting expectations about treatment modalities, priorities, and outcomes of health care services including health promotion activities (Hornsten et al., 2004).

In developing sustainable health promotion programs, examination of health behaviors and the determinants of health behaviors provide an important foundation for identifying factors related to active participation in health promotion programs. Individuals' health behaviors are better illustrated when examined within the context of their conceptualization of health (Laffrey, 1986; Pender, 1987). For example, if individuals do not perceive the importance or the relationship of different dimensions of health to health status, they may not embrace lifestyle behaviors that enhance health status. What we think about health comes from our own point of view with our minds and bodies working together to keep us healthy.

Health conceptualization studies across persons with a variety of disabilities have shown multidimensional views concerning the concept of health that parallel those of their peers without disabilities (e.g., eating healthy foods, being physically able to do things, having relationships, not being in pain, being able to deal with negative remarks, being able to express thoughts, having plenty of people who love you, doing things for yourself). But individuals with disabilities also incorporate their own life experiences as persons who have disabilities and/or health conditions (Marks, 1996). For example, a person with DD may say the following: "I'm healthy when I use my wheelchair" or "I'm not healthy when I'm not using my wheelchair," and "I'm healthy when I take my pills for my diabetes" or "I'm healthy when I don't have to take pills." Adults with disabilities may also state that they are healthy even though they have a chronic condition or disability (Marks, 1996).

In general, definitions of health can be viewed from several different domains. For example, some people feel healthy when they are not sick. They may think of physical definitions, such as having no aches or pains, feeling strong, or not having any illness or disease. These definitions are used to define *physical health*. Other people define health using a *social health* definition. They will say that they are healthy when they feel comfortable where they live and work and have close relationships with others. Health can also be defined using an *emotional* definition of health. Emotional definitions of health can include things such as liking yourself, being able to do the things that you want to do, or handling stressful events. *Spiritual health* can also be used to define health. Spiritual health definitions include feelings of satisfaction, happiness, and sense of purpose with life. Finally, some people also define being healthy using an *intellectual health* definition, which includes an ability to learn and use knowledge.

Understanding health conceptualizations of people with disabilities is imperative because disability is a natural part of the human experience. Like people addressing race and gender issues, individuals with disabilities are disentangling socially constructed determinants from those attributable to physiology. They are identifying as members of a sociocultural group across diagnostic boundaries and viewing social, political, and economic barriers as a large part of daily concerns (Gill, 1987). What health means to us can depend on our needs, goals, and life experiences, as well as where we live, work, and have fun. For individuals with disabilities, health concepts may differ from their peers without disabilities due to differences in physical, social, cognitive, and emotional abilities. But, like their peers without disabilities, adults with disabilities may also feel healthy when they have fun with their family and friends.

Life Expectancy for Adults with Disabilities

Adults with intellectual and developmental disabilities (I/DD) were estimated to make up 1.5% of the noninstitutionalized population in the early 2000s (DelParigi et al., 2002; Larson et al., 2001). By 2030, the number of adults with I/DD over the age of 60 years is expected to nearly double from 641,860 to an estimated 1.2 million (Yamaki & Fujiura, 2002). Improvements in medicine and standards of living provide people with DD an opportunity to live longer.

Across all types of disabilities, the life expectancy for people with disabilities acquired early in life has increased significantly. However, in general, people with disabilities have a life expectancy that is 15–20 years less than the rest of the population. With advances in medical treatment and living conditions, life expectancy for some people with disabilities (e.g., people with spinal cord injury) has risen dramatically and is only slightly lower than that of the general population. For people with Down syndrome, cerebral palsy (particularly for individuals with lower levels of functioning), and severe intellectual disabilities, life expectancy is significantly lower than for the general population (Bittles, Bower, Hussain, & Glasson, 2002; Janicki, Dalton, Henderson, & Davidson, 1999; Patja, Iivanainen, Vesala, Oksanen, & Ruoppila, 2000). In addition, life expectancy for individuals with DD is significantly lower than that of the general population in the presence of the following impairments: severe mobility impairment (requiring a wheelchair and assistance for propulsion), severe manual dexterity impairment (unable to feed and dress without assistance), and severe intellectual disability (intelligence quotient [IQ] < 50).

How Adults with Disabilities Age

People with disabilities may age differently based on the nature and severity of their disability, coexisting health conditions, and chronic health conditions. Several issues may have an impact on morbidity and mortality for people with DD, such as chronic respiratory infections, heart conditions, reduced mobility, epilepsy and refractory seizures, dependency in eating and toileting, and severe and profound intellectual disabilities. Cardiovascular disease is one of the most common causes of death among aging adults with DD (Beange, McElduff, & Baker, 1995; Draheim, 2006; Haveman, 2007; Iacono & Sutherland, 2006; Yamaki, 2005). Data also demonstrate higher rates of obesity and poor nutritional habits among adults with DD compared with the general population (Fujiura, Fitzsimons, Marks, & Chicoine, 1997; Rimmer & Yamaki, 2006; Sisirak, Marks, Heller, & Riley, 2007; Yamaki, 2005).

The unique needs of adults with DD across the lifespan present opportunities for health care professionals to develop health systems aimed at supporting them to achieve optimal health status. How well adults with DD age in later life depends on their health behaviors throughout their lifetime. Outcomes of aging well may consist of 1) living on one's own terms; 2) adding value to society, family, and/or friends; and 3) having control over determinants of health through health promotion activities and supportive environments. Many of the problems associated with normal aging are attributed to a "high-risk lifestyle." Hence, health promotion and disease prevention activities are seen as a way to age well by lowering the risk for disease and illness later in life.

Health Concerns for Individuals with Developmental Disabilities

Individuals with DD who have lived 30–50 years with disabilities are experiencing new health concerns, and many people now aging with disabilities experience a multitude of premature medical, functional, and psychosocial problems as they age. Long-term disabilities are often not stable over the lifespan, and an aging gap is becoming evident as many individuals with disabilities experience functional changes that are customarily not seen in people without disabilities until much later in life. Although disentangling the impact of disability, aging, and the combination of aging with a disability on various health concerns is difficult, evidence suggests that people with DD do experience age-related health conditions earlier, including incontinence, swallowing difficulties, sensory losses, adaptive behavior losses, and cognitive declines (Janicki et al., 2002; Prasher, 1995). Adults with DD may also experience an increase in chronic conditions related to altered postures, immobility, long-term use of medications, and poor nutrition.

> *Many people now aging with disabilities experience a multitude of premature* medical, functional, and psychosocial problems as they age.

Health Outcomes and Contributing Factors for Adults with Developmental Disabilities

Health outcomes can vary among groups of people based on age and socioeconomic status. In general, essential requirements for health include food, housing, education, income, sustainable resources, social justice, equity, and peace (World Health Organization [WHO], 2001a). Major determinants of preventable illness and death are often the result of inadequate and poor health literacy skills, limited social support, poverty, and unemployment (not just physiological and psychological factors). Determinants of health status can be categorized into four broad areas: 1) biological factors (e.g., syndrome and gender-related conditions), 2) socioeconomic and environmental factors, 3) access to health care (e.g., physical, communication, and programmatic aspects), and 4) behavioral factors (e.g., lifestyle choices, health promotion/disease prevention practices) (Tarlov, 1996). To improve health or to modify conditions for people with DD, consideration of these four areas must be addressed in order to achieve successful results. Figure 1.1 presents the multiple influences on health for persons with disabilities.

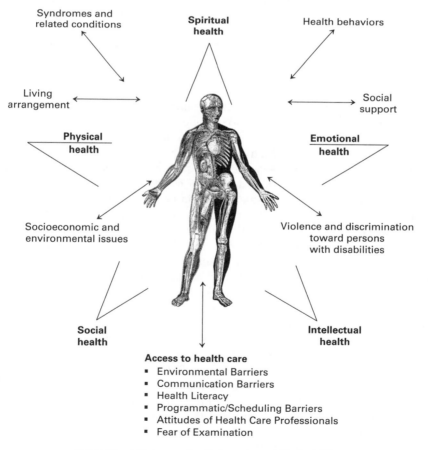

Figure 1.1. Influence on health for persons with disabilities.

Biological Factors (Syndromes and Gender)

Individuals with DD who have syndrome-related conditions are predisposed to a myriad of health conditions based on their type of disability, making health promotion and disease prevention activities critical. For example, people aging with cerebral palsy (CP) may have increased problems related to bowel and bladder issues that are associated with urinary tract infections, respiratory disease and infections (leading cause of death), difficulty eating or swallowing, dental problems, reduced mobility, bone demineralization, fractures, fatigue, gastroesophageal reflux, spasticity, pain, arthritis, decreased muscle tone, musculoskeletal deformities, decreased ambulation, and progressive cervical spine degeneration (White-Scott, 2007).

People aging with CP and epilepsy who use psychotropic and antiseizure medications on a long-term basis also have a higher risk of developing osteoporosis (i.e., brittle bone disease) and tardive dyskinesia (i.e., repetitive, involuntary, purposeless movements caused by the long-term use of certain drugs). This risk is often compounded by limited physical activity and diets limited in calcium and vitamin D. Antiepileptic medications are also frequently given long term to individuals with DD. Studies suggest that osteoporosis and osteomalacia (i.e., softening of the bones) are potential side effects of certain antiepileptic medication, and vitamin D levels may be reduced leading to possible loss of bone mass. Other medications can induce liver enzymes that interfere with the metabolism of vitamin D and calcium, which is essential for bone health.

Adults with Down syndrome have a higher prevalence of early-onset Alzheimer's disease (15% to 40%) compared with the general population, and they experience hypothyroidism and sleep apnea more frequently (McCarron, Gill, McCallion, & Begley, 2005). Having Down syndrome also predisposes people to certain types of health conditions, such as congenital heart disease, hypotonia or low muscle tone, eye conditions, cervical spine conditions, hypotension or low blood pressure, low heart rate, thyroid disease, weight issues, seizures, early menopause, and osteoporosis (Beange et al., 1995; Freeman et al., 1998). Adults with Down syndrome are also at a greater risk for joint problems, tumors, and leukemia (Freeman et al., 1998). In addition, limited research suggests that adults with Down syndrome residing in community-based settings have elevated risk factors for cardiovascular disease, such as hypercholesterolemia (high cholesterol), hypertriglyceridemia (high triglycerides), elevated fasting insulin levels, abdominal obesity, and a high prevalence of undiagnosed non-insulin dependent diabetes mellitus (Draheim, McCubbin, & Williams, 2002).

Aging adults with fragile X syndrome may have more issues with heart problems, musculoskeletal disorder, earlier menopause in women, epilepsy, and visual problems (Prasher & Janicki, 2002). High rates of cardiovascular disease; diabetes; appetite disorders; sleep disturbances; respiratory concerns; and weight management issues and other obesity-related problems such as hypoventilation, hypertension, right-sided heart failure, stasis ulcers, cellulitis, and skin problems in fat folds, are seen in people with Prader-Willi syndrome.

Men and women also experience different conditions based on gender. To illustrate, whereas men are diagnosed with breast cancer, the prevalence rate is much lower compared with women. Also, women are more likely to have osteoporosis and depression (Walsh, 2002).

Socioeconomic and Environmental Issues

Socioeconomic and environmental factors affect health status. Where people live, work, and play matters. For example, obesity rates in the general population vary by different regions in the country. Figure 1.2 depicts the percentage of obesity in states across the country (Centers for Disease Control and Prevention, n.d.; National Center for Chronic Disease Prevention and Health Promotion, 2007).

For adults with DD, living in specific residential settings and participating in day programs (i.e., work sites) can affect health status (Rimmer, Braddock, & Marks, 1995). Adults living in the community have the highest rates of obesity. Also, individuals with particular syndromes, such as Down syndrome, have a higher prevalence of being overweight and obese.

Limited social support, along with disruption of personal ties, loneliness, violence directed at individuals with disabilities, and conflicted interactions with peers and caregivers, can be major sources of stress for adults with DD. Inadequate social support is associated with an increase in mortality, morbidity, and psychological distress and a decrease in overall general health. Supportive social connections and intimate relations are vital sources of emotional strength and have a positive effect on health status.

Currently, families are the major providers of care for adults with DD (see Figure 1.3). More than 76% of adults of all ages with DD live with their families (Braddock, 1999; Fujiura, 2003). As people with DD have the opportunity to live longer, their parents may experience extended caregiving responsibilities at a time in life when they are experiencing their own health care issues and are potentially

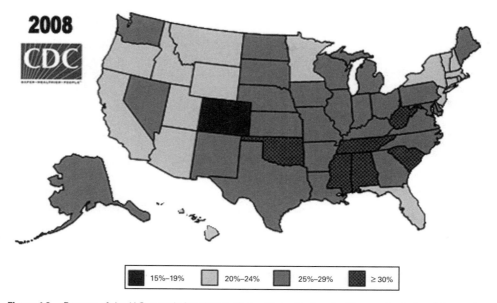

Figure 1.2. Percent of the U.S. population that is obese. (From Centers for Disease Control and Prevention [CDC, 2008a]. *Behavioral Risk Factor Surveillance System Survey Data.* Atlanta, Georgia: U.S. Department of Health and Human Services, Centers for Disease Control and Prevention. Available at http://www.cdc.gov/obesity/data/trends.html#State).

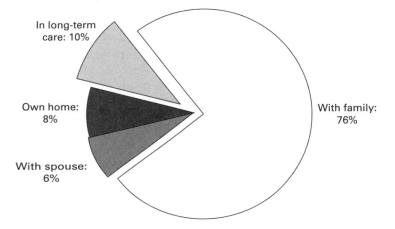

Figure 1.3. Where do people live? Living arrangements of people with developmental disabilities, by percentage, according to a national health interview survey. (*Source:* Fujiura, 1998)

in need of caregiver support for themselves. More than 25% of families supporting a child or other relative in the home are headed by adults age 60 years or older (Braddock, Hemp, & Rizzolo 2008), and another 38% are headed by adults between the ages of 41 and 59 years. Few family support services are available for families and they also face long waiting lists for residential services (Prouty, Smith, & Lakin, 2006). Many service delivery systems and communities are not prepared to meet the needs of adults with DD who will likely need day and residential services as they age and no longer have parents to provide care for them.

> *Supportive social connections and intimate relations are vital sources of emotional strength and have a positive effect on health status.*

In addition to receiving support from families, many adults with DD also received support from a community-based organization (CBO). About 56% of adults with DD participate in day- and/or work-segregated services including day programs, day habilitation, clinic, or rehabilitation. This provides a greater opportunity for CBOs to reach out to individuals with DD who are most likely living with their families (Braddock et al., 2008).

Access to Health Care

Adults with disabilities face challenges when attempting to obtain social and health services. Because of different developmental trajectories and limitations in communication and cognitive skills, health care delivery to people with DD is often ineffective or absent (Beange et al., 1995), and the result is underdiagnosis, misdiagnosis, or less chance of receiving prompt treatment.

Access barriers (e.g., programmatic, attitudinal, physical, communication, and limited health literacy skill) and inadequate professional education regarding disability issues frequently are not addressed in health care services (see Table 1.1). Although many Americans face obstacles to obtaining health care, primarily related to health insurance issues, people with DD are especially vulnerable to the inade-

Table 1.1. Access barriers to health services

Programmatic barriers	Includes inflexible appointments that fail to accommodate transportation difficulties, underinsured or no health insurance coverage, geographic unavailability of health services, and/or lack of assistance in examination rooms
Attitudinal barriers	Experienced by people with disabilities when health professionals lack knowledge and sensitivities about disabilities. Specific issues relate to diagnostic overshadowing (i.e., an overfocus on the disability-related issues leads to overlooking new or emerging health conditions that may be present) and treating an individual as a "diagnosis" and not as a person.
Physical barriers	Includes inaccessible examination tables (e.g., too high or low to transfer from a wheelchair), inaccessible restrooms, lack of signage regarding accessible entrances, and lack of braille signage in facility
Communication barriers	May prevent people with visual, hearing, and/or learning disabilities from receiving information in an understandable format. For example, inappropriate presentation of teaching materials, such as the lack of sign interpreters, large print formats for health education materials, and materials that are appropriate for level of intellectual functioning, may inhibit learning.
Limited health literacy skills	May prevent people from gaining control over their health and managing chronic conditions. *Early* and *lifelong* health education is a critical component for people to increase health literacy skills.
Fear of examination	May prevent people from getting the health treatment that they need

quacies of the existing health care system. Moreover, they share experiences similar to racial/ethnic minorities related to marginalization, poverty, abuse, and lack of support, which reduce access to health education, preventive health screenings, and health promotion activities (Gill, 1996; Kopack, Fritz, & Holt, 1996).

Unfortunately, many health care providers have not had the necessary training or experience to provide health care services for adults with DD (Lennox, Diggens, & Ugoni, 1997; Phillips, Morrison, & Davis, 2004). Moreover, individuals with DD report that health care professionals often lack knowledge and sensitivities about their disabilities and focus more on their disabilities rather than on their immediate health problems (Gill, 1997). Professionals also tend to objectify people with disabilities as a "diagnosis" or "disease" that needs to be cured (or fixed), a perspective that fails to see them as healthy and able to benefit from health promotion and self-care activities. This perspective further alienates and marginalizes adults with DD and lessens their chances for obtaining and engaging in health promoting services. Accessing services may also be difficult due to the refusal of a person with a disability to be examined or to professionals' refusal to provide services (Gill, 1997).

As health system resources decrease, the increased time pressures for health care providers are especially problematic for adults with DD who often need extra time for examinations, tests, procedures, and communication. Health care providers need to be prepared to provide more information about

> *Although many Americans face obstacles to obtaining health care, people with DD are especially vulnerable to the inadequacies of the existing health care system.*

routine and specialized treatment and health maintenance to make people with DD comfortable and help them make informed health care choices. Educating caregivers about health-related issues is one strategy that can be used to achieve increased understanding of health information among people with DD (Marks & Heller, 2003).

Access to Health Care for Women with Developmental Disabilities

Women with DD often do not receive appropriate access to health care. Many times, women with DD do not receive information on developmental changes and safe sexual practices (Heller & Marks, 2002), and women living in community-based settings are less likely than their peers without disabilities to receive preventive health screenings (e.g., mammography and Pap smear) that would reduce disparities in health status (Heller & Marks, 2002). Lack of adherence to preventive screenings by women with DD may be related to low income, low educational level, lack of continuity with health care providers, reluctance to be seen by male physicians, lack of adapted equipment, lack of health insurance coverage, and difficulty in arranging examinations (Heller & Marks, 2002).

For these women, supportive environments enable them to engage in health promotion and disease-prevention activities. Health promotion consists of screening activities to decrease the risk of acquiring a specific health condition or early detection of a particular condition (e.g., more women would be screened for breast and cervical cancer if their doctors recommended these screenings). Lack of adapted equipment may prevent women with musculoskeletal disabilities from receiving preventive health screening. For women, routine health visits need to include the following screenings: breast cancer, cervical cancer, and osteoporosis. Also, screening for depression is recommended because women with DD have high rates of depression, which is often undetected (Lunsky & Havercamp, 2002).

Health Behaviors

Behavioral factors of health include getting adequate exercise, practicing good nutritional habits, refraining from smoking, and understanding options and choices regarding decision making (Marks & Heller, 2003). Health behaviors can directly influence health status for adults with DD and may indirectly affect health by influencing environmental factors. Removing or modifying behavioral risk factors associated with the acceleration of disease processes can postpone the development of common chronic diseases. In general, health behaviors maintain or enhance health status, control or remove harmful risk factors, and prevent the onset of chronic conditions.

Although genetics and environmental toxins can influence the development of chronic disease, poor health behaviors are the primary contributor to chronic disease for most people (Grantmakers Health, 2004). More than 90 million Americans live with chronic diseases, and every year, more than 1.7 million people die from them (Centers for Disease Control and Prevention, 2008b). Chronic conditions, such as heart disease, cancer, lung disease, stroke, and diabetes, are among the most common. Susan Curry (Grantmakers Health, 2004, p. 1) stated, "The top three actual causes of death in the United States are behaviorally related... All told, modifiable lifestyle factors account for about half of premature deaths in the United States."

Dietary intake and physical activity patterns are major determinants of being overweight and being obese (World Health Organization, 2003). For the general population and for adults with DD, the combination of sedentary lifestyles, high fat diets, and low fruit and vegetable diets is a major contributor to increased risk for acquiring chronic health conditions.

Health Literacy

The Surgeon General's *Call to Action to Improve the Health and Wellness of Persons with Disabilities* (U.S. Department of Health and Human Services, 2005b) noted the following challenges related to health-related communication:

1. Providers are unprepared to engage in dialogue and shared decision making and are uncomfortable with (or lack knowledge in) discussing disabilities.

2. Much of everyday health information has not incorporated principles of universal design (i.e., barrier-free or accessible design) for individuals with DD.

3. Patients and/or caregivers often do not have or think they do not have enough information.

4. Cross-cultural gaps exist between providers, individuals with DD, and caregivers.

In developing accessible health promotion services for individuals with DD, health care providers, support people, and individuals with DD themselves increasingly share responsibility for health-related decisions. People with DD and their care providers need to develop specific skills to improve literacy related to health issues; families, community-service providers, and health services providers need to increase clear health communication using multimodal strategies to ensure accessibility. Frameworks for understanding health literacy issues among individuals with DD throughout their lifespan must incorporate definitions of health literacy, components of clear communication, and the central role of health literacy skills and communication capacities among individuals with DD and their caregivers.

Health literacy is defined as the degree to which individuals have the capacity to obtain, process, and understand basic health information and services needed to make appropriate health decisions (Selden, Zorn, Ratzan, & Parker, 2000). This definition has evolved from a passive role for individuals to a comprehensive, holistic definition that encourages active participation in making informed health care decisions—more than just being able to read pamphlets and make appointments (Ad Hoc Committee on Health Literacy for the Council on Scientific Affairs: American Medical Association, 1999; U.S. Department of Health and Human Services, 2000; World Health Organization, 1998).

Research demonstrates the influence of health literacy on health outcomes. Individuals with low health literacy have higher utilization of treatment services, increased hospitalization and emergency services, and lower utilization of preventive services, resulting in higher health care costs. Another critical component of health literacy is its impact on people's ability to navigate the health care system, including locating providers and services and filling out forms. In the general population, only 12% of adults have proficient health literacy (Baur, 2007; National Center for Education Statistics, 2003). Put another way, 9 out of 10 adults may lack the skills needed to manage their health and prevent disease.

Improving health literacy requires attention to both system and individual level factors. Although everyone may not be able to read or remember when to take his or her medication, systems can be put in place to support participation in health care, such as pictures or cues for remembering what his or her medications look like and when to take them (Zarcadoolas, Pleasant, & Greer, 2006). Individual level factors that affect health literacy include communication skills of lay people and professionals, knowledge of lay people and professionals of health topics, culture, demands of the health care and public health systems, and demands of the situation/context (Baur, 2007). Health literacy depends on lay person and professional knowledge of various health topics. People with limited or inaccurate knowledge about the body and the causes of disease may not understand the relationship between lifestyle factors (e.g., diet, exercise) and health outcomes or recognize when they need to seek care. The negative health consequences of low health literacy skills may be even greater among individuals with disabilities and other minority populations, including individuals with limited English proficiency as well as older adults, those who are financially impoverished, and people with limited education.

Health literacy can be an approach for empowering an individual to express his or her own health concerns, which is critical in gaining control over one's own health (Freire, 1972; World Health Organization, 1998). Having health literacy skills allows people to share personal and health information with health care providers; engage in self-care and chronic disease management; adopt health-promoting behaviors, such as exercising and eating a healthy diet; and act on health-related news and announcements. In turn, these outcomes affect health status, health care costs, and quality of care. According to the Institute of Medicine Committee on Health Care in America's *Crossing the Quality Chasm: A New Health System for the 21st Century*, "Good quality means providing patients with appropriate services, in a technically competent manner, with good communication, shared decision making, and cultural sensitivity" (2001, p. 232). Although early detection of disease risk may help to reduce such disparities, many adults with DD do not participate in preventive health care at recommended levels (Iacono & Sutherland, 2006). In addition, adults with DD frequently have not been taught how to accurately communicate early signs and symptoms of chronic conditions to their health care providers, which is problematic in being able to understand and follow treatment recommendations.

> *People with limited or inaccurate knowledge about the body and the causes of disease may not understand the relationship between lifestyle factors and health outcomes or recognize when they need to seek care.*

The provision of health information in an accessible format is a critical ingredient for adults with DD to gain knowledge and understanding about health issues and their bodies, along with ways they can take charge of their health. However, limited research on access to health care for adults with DD (primarily qualitative designs) suggests that key issues include poor communication skills of general practitioners and other primary care staff, problems in getting appointment times or home visits, and crowded surgery waiting rooms (Turk & Burchell, 2003). For people with DD, more information is needed to reduce their fears and to help them make informed health care choices. As health care providers and patients increasingly share responsibility for treatment decisions, people with DD need the opportunity to develop specific skills to become literate in health care issues, and providers need to increase clear health communication using multimodal strategies (e.g., visual, written, verbal, tactile).

Obesity

Obesity is defined as excess body fat accumulation caused by increased energy input and decreased energy output (Bray, 1987). Obesity has become one of the most prevalent health conditions in the United States with more than half of American adults being classified as either overweight or obese (Hedley et al., 2004; Ogden et al., 2006). According to the U.S. Surgeon General, rates of people who are overweight and rates of people who are obese have reached epidemic proportions, contributing to 300,000 deaths in the United States per year (U.S. Department of Health and Human Services, 2001). Since the late 1990s, obesity rates have increased by more than 20% (Newby et al., 2003). The most recent data from the 2003–2004 National Health and Nutrition Examination Survey estimate the prevalence of both people who are overweight and people who are obese combined at 66%, and the prevalence of obesity alone was at 32.2% among adults in the general population (Ogden et al., 2006). Excess weight is recognized as a risk factor in more than 45 diseases and health conditions, specifically contributing to heart disease, diabetes, stroke, hypertension, arthritis, certain cancers, stress, depression, and respiratory problems (Chan, Rimm, Colditz, Stampfer, & Willett, 1994; Colditz, Willett, Rotnitzky, & Manson, 1995; Eckel, 1997; Haffner & Taegtmeyer, 2003; Hubert, Feinleib, McNamara, & Castelli, 1983; Must et al., 1999; National Heart Lung and Blood Institute's Obesity Education Initiative, 1995; National Task Force on the Prevention and Treatment of Obesity, 2000; Pi-Sunyer, 1999; Sturm & Wells, 2001).

The prevalence of overweight and obese adults with DD has been estimated to be either equal or higher compared with the general population (Harris, Rosenberg, Jangda, O'Brien, & Gallagher, 2003; Jansen, Krol, Groothoff, & Post, 2004; Melville, Hamilton, Hankey, Miller, & Boyle, 2006; Rimmer & Yamaki, 2006; Rubin, Rimmer, Chicoine, Braddock, & McGuire, 1998; Yamaki, 2005). Yamaki (2005), in the first U.S. population-based study of adults with intellectual and developmental disabilities (I/DD), reported a combined prevalence of overweight and obesity at 63.5% and the prevalence of obesity alone at 34.6%. Over the past several decades, maintaining a healthy weight decreased for adults with DD with the overall percentage of healthy weight in adults with I/DD decreasing from 48% in 1985–1988 to 34% in 1997–2000. Refer to Table 1.2 and Figures 1.4–1.6 for more information about obesity among adults with DD and in the general population.

Rates of being overweight or obese are reportedly higher in people living in community-based settings (Frey & Rimmer, 1995; Lewis, Lewis, Leake, King, & Lindemann, 2002; Prasher, 1995; Rimmer, Braddock, & Fujiura, 1993; Rimmer et al., 1995; Rimmer & Yamaki, 2006; Rubin et al., 1998; van Schrojenstein & Valk, 2005), individuals with higher levels of cognitive functioning (Rimmer et al., 1993), women, older adults (Yamaki, 2005), and people with specific genetic syndromes such as Down syndrome and Prader-Willi (Bell & Bhate, 1992; Fujiura et al., 1997;

Table 1.2.   Prevalence of obesity (by percent) among adults with intellectual and developmental disabilities (I/DD)

Prevalence	1985–1988	1997–2000
	%	%
Total		
Adults with I/DD	19	35
General population	11	21
Sex		
Men with I/DD	18	27
Men in general population	11	20
Women with I/DD	22	44
Women in general population	12	21
Age		
18–39 with I/DD	19	34
18–39 in general population	9	17
40–65 with I/DD	20	36
40–65 in general population	15	24

Source: Yamaki (2005).

Prasher, 1995; Rimmer & Wang, 2005; Rimmer & Yamaki, 2006; Rubin et al., 1998). Adults with DD who live in community-based settings also tend to have low fitness levels and lead sedentary lifestyles (Melville et al., 2006; Rimmer & Yamaki, 2006; Rubin et al., 1998; Yamaki, 2005). For individuals with DD, the combination of sedentary lifestyles, high-fat diets, and low fruit and vegetable intake increases their susceptibility to health conditions, such as obesity, cardiovascular disease (CVD), osteoporosis, hypertension, Type II diabetes, and depression (Beange et al., 1995; Draheim, Williams, & McCubbin, 2002; Fujiura et al., 1997; Rimmer & Yamaki, 2006; Yamaki, 2005). CVD is one of the most common causes of death among adults with I/DD (Hayden, 1998; Janicki et al., 1999). The onset of CVD is strongly associated with lack of physical activity and poor nutrition (Prasher, 1995; Rimmer et al., 1995; Rimmer & Yamaki, 2006; Robertson et al., 2000).

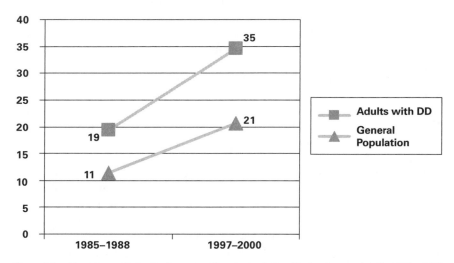

Figure 1.4.   Prevalence of obesity (by percent) among adults with developmental disabilities (DD) and the general population. (*Source:* Yamaki, 2005)

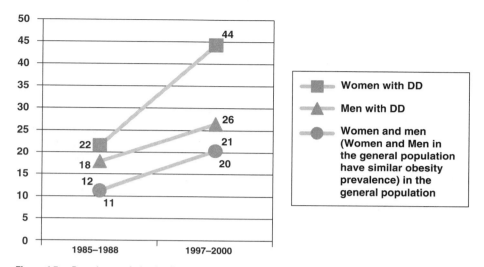

Figure 1.5. Prevalence of obesity (by percent) among adults with developmental disabilities (DD) by gender. (*Source:* Yamaki, 2005)

Changing the Course:
Investing in Health Promotion

Investing in health promotion activities for people with disabilities can have a substantial impact on improving health and reducing the personal and financial costs associated with poor health. In the United States, diet and physical activity patterns are driving the current epidemic of overweight and obesity.

The combination of sedentary lifestyles, high-fat diets, and low fruit and vegetable intake increases susceptibility to health conditions.

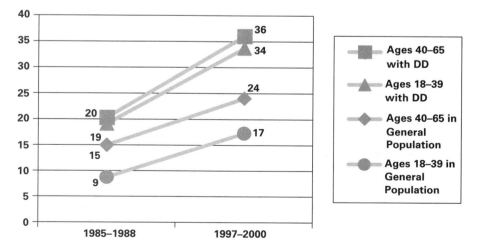

Figure 1.6. Prevalence of obesity (by percent) among adults with developmental disabilities (DD) by age. (*Source:* Yamaki, 2005)

Physically inactive people are almost twice as likely to develop heart disease as active people (American Heart Association, 2010). This makes inactivity as strong of a risk factor for heart disease as smoking, high blood pressure, or high cholesterol.

Chronic health conditions are at least one underlying cause for increased health problems and associated expenditures for people with disabilities. In the general population, decades of health promotion research have documented that high risk employees cost more and are less productive. Research has also documented the benefits of worksite health promotion programs on reducing health risks, decreasing medical and disability claims, and lowering absenteeism. Comprehensive health promotion programs have a positive return on investment (Aldana, 1998; Anderson et al., 2000; Burton, Conti, Chen, Schultz, & Edington, 1999; Edington, Yen, & Witting, 1997; Fries, Harrington, Edwards, Kent, & Richardson, 1994; Goetzel et al., 1998; Goetzel, Juday, & Ozminkowski, 1999; Gold, Anderson, & Serxner, 2000; Pelletier, 1999; Serxner, Gold, Anderson, & Williams, 2001; Wood, Olmstead, & Craig, 1989). Unfortunately, health promotion for individuals with disabilities has lagged decades behind the health promotion movement for their peers without disabilities.

In December 2002, the Surgeon General held a conference on Health Disparities and Mental Retardation to address growing concerns about the health status of individuals with I/DD. This conference resulted in the *Closing the Gap: National Blueprint to Improve the Health of Persons with Mental Retardation* report, which identified a primary goal aimed at integrating "health promotion into community environments of people with mental retardation." Since this report, the term *mental retardation* is no longer in common use and has been replaced by the term *intellectual and developmental disabilities*. A second goal in this report aimed to increase knowledge and understanding of health through practical and useful information (U.S. Public Health Service, 2002).

Physical Activity, Exercise, and Fitness

Understanding the differences between physical activity and fitness is one of the first steps in developing a health promotion program for individuals with DD. *Physical activity* is typically seen as any form of exercise or movement. *Fitness* is defined as planned exercise using standard guidelines with the goal of changing body composition in targeted areas that include the following: flexibility, aerobic endurance (cardiovascular endurance), balance, and muscle strength (National Institute of Diabetes and Digestive Kidney Diseases, 2007).

Physical activity may include planned activity, such as walking, running, basketball, or other sports. It may also include other daily activities, such as household chores, yard work, or walking the dog (National Institute of Diabetes and Digestive Kidney Diseases, 2007). In general, both fitness activity and physical activity are important when attempting to change attitudes and perceptions of people who are not currently physically active. Individuals will see more physical changes with regular fitness activity than with physical activity.

Physical Activity and Adults with Developmental Disabilities: How Much Do They Actually Do? Approximately 10% of adults with DD engage in physical activity a minimum of 3 days per week, compared with about 15% of adults in the general population. Up to 50% of adults with DD engage in no exercise

compared with 25% of adults in the general population (Centers for Disease Control and Prevention, Division of Nutrition, 2008). One study found that less than 1% of adults with I/DD participated in regular, vigorous activity three times per week. Most leisure-time activities are sedentary, such as watching television or listening to the radio (Frey, Buchanan, & Sandt, 2005; Melville et al., 2007; Rimmer & Yamaki, 2006).

What Keeps Adults with Developmental Disabilities from Exercising?

Caregivers and adults with DD have different perceptions about the knowledge and the skills needed to exercise. Individuals with DD will exercise more if their caregivers believe that exercise will benefit them and if they have fewer access barriers (Heller, Hsieh, & Rimmer, 2004; Heller, Ying, Rimmer, & Marks, 2002). In addition, it is important for caregivers to understand 1) their own expectations and perceptions of barriers related to exercise for people with disabilities, and 2) people with disabilities's expectations and perceptions of barriers relating to exercise. Research has shown that adults with DD and their caregiver informants report different benefits (or outcome expectations towards exercising). Table 1.3 compares outcome expectations toward exercising (Heller et al., 2004).

Adults with DD and their caregivers also report different barriers (access barriers and cognitive-emotional barriers). In a study conducted by the University of Illinois at Chicago's (UIC's) Health Promotion Program, at baseline more than 66% of participants with I/DD reported receiving little support for exercising, and more than 50% lacked confidence to perform exercise (Heller et al., 2004). Adults with DD and their caregivers reported several key barriers to exercise:

- Cost

- Being tired or bored by exercising

- Problems with using equipment

- Lack of energy

- Transportation issues

- No one to show them how to exercise

- Concern that people might make fun of them

Table 1.3. Outcome expectations toward exercising: Persons with developmental disabilities (DD) and their staff informants

Outcome expectations	Persons with DD (%)	Informants (%)
Lose or control body weight	80	73
Give more energy	30	73**
Make body feel good physically	75	80
Make mind feel good emotionally	89	75
Decrease joint pain and stiffness	36	52*
Meet new people	64	68
Get in shape	77	82
Look better	89	73
Improve overall health	80	91

McNemar statistical tests: *$p<.05$, **$p<.01$

- Exercise being too difficult

- Lack of accessible fitness centers

Despite reporting a variety of barriers to exercising, adults with DD and their staff differed on which barriers were the most problematic. Tables 1.4 and 1.5 compare perceptions of access and cognitive-emotional barriers between individuals with DD and their staff. In Tables 1.3, 1.4, and 1.5, the differences in expectations and perceptions between individuals with DD and their informants are shown. In these tables, the value of .01 means that there is a 99% (1 – .01 = .99) chance of the difference between participant and informant being true; the value of .001 means that there is a 99.9% (1 – .001 = .999) chance of the difference between participant and informant being true.

For example, in Table 1.3, the expectations toward exercising that differed the most related to energy and joint pain. With regard to energy, 30% of people with DD expected to have more energy with exercising compared with 73% of their staff informants; and 52% of staff informants thought that the individuals with disabilities would have less joint pain and stiffness compared with 36% of people with disabilities (Heller et al., 2004).

In Table 1.4, the access barriers relating to exercising that differed the most were costs, concern that people would make fun of them, and lack of instruction. In regard to costs, 25% of people with DD thought that it was too expensive to exercise compared with 9% of their staff informants, 2% of staff informants had concern that people would make fun of them compared with 41% of individuals with disabilities, and 2% of staff informants had concern that no one would show them how to exercise compared with 34% individuals with disabilities (Heller et al., 2004).

> In a health promotion study, 25% of people with I/DD thought that it was too expensive to exercise, and 41% thought it was too difficult to exercise.

The cognitive-emotional barriers in Table 1.5 relating to exercising that differed the most were level of difficulty and health concerns. Forty-one percent of people with DD thought that it was too difficult to exercise compared with 14% of their staff informants, and 14% of staff informants thought that health concerns prevented

Table 1.4. Perceptions of access barriers to exercising: Persons with developmental disabilities (DD) and their staff informants

Access barriers	Persons with DD (%)	Informants (%)
Costs too much	25	9*
Transportation not available	21	36
Don't know how	46	25
Don't know where	39	21
No one to exercise with	11	14
Equipment hard to use	11	5
People might make fun of them	41	2**
No one to show them how to exercise	34	2**
Inaccessible fitness centers	30	25

McNemar statistical test: *percentage <.05, **percentage <.001

Table 1.5. Perceptions of cognitive-emotional barriers to exercising: Persons with developmental disabilities (DD) and their staff informants

Cognitive-emotional barriers	Persons with DD (%)	Informants (%)
Lack of time	25	39
Lack of interest	21	34
Lack of energy	46	21
Boring	39	34
Not improving condition	11	25
Making condition worse	11	9
Too difficult	41	14*
Health concerns	34	14*
Too lazy	30	23

McNemar statistical tests: *$p < .05$

people with disabilities from exercising compared with 34% of individuals with disabilities (Heller et al., 2004).

How Much Physical Activity Should Adults with Developmental Disabilities Do?
Current recommendations state that vigorous exercise is not necessary to obtain health benefits. Moderate intensity activities, such as walking, swimming, dancing, and gentle exercise can result in improved health and well-being (see Table 1.6 for examples of exercises that require moderate amounts of activity). It is recommended that adults get at least 30 minutes of moderate physical activity most days of the week. Moderate physical activity is any activity that requires about as much energy as walking 2 miles in 30 minutes.

U.S. Department of Agriculture Guidelines for Physical Activity
The U.S. Department of Agriculture (USDA) *Dietary Guidelines for Americans 2005* have provided recommendations for physical activity. These recommendations are listed next (http://www.health.gov/dietaryguidelines/dga2005/recommendations. htm):

Table 1.6. Examples of moderate amounts of physical activities

Basketball (playing a game) for 15–20 minutes	Running 1½ miles in 15 minutes (10 minutes per mile)
Basketball (shooting baskets) for 30 minutes	Shoveling snow for 15 minutes
Bicycling 4 miles in 15 minutes	Stairwalking for 15 minutes
Bicycling 5 miles in 30 minutes	Swimming laps for 20 minutes
Dancing fast (social) for 30 minutes	Walking 1¾ miles in 35 minutes (20 minutes per mile)
Gardening for 30–45 minutes	Walking 2 miles in 30 minutes (15 minutes per mile)
Jumping rope for 15 minutes	Washing and waxing a car for 45–60 minutes
Playing touch football for 30–45 minutes	Washing windows or floors for 45–60 minutes
Playing volleyball for 45 minutes	Water aerobics for 30 minutes
Pushing a stroller 1½ miles in 30 minutes	Wheelchair basketball for 20 minutes
Raking leaves for 30 minutes	Wheeling self in wheelchair for 30–40 minutes

From National Heart, Lung, and Blood Institute. (2010) *Guide to physical activity.* Available from http://www.nhlbi.nih.gov/health/public/heart/obesity/lose_wt/phy_act.htm

- Engage in regular physical activity and reduce sedentary activities to promote health, psychological well-being, and a healthy body weight.
    - To reduce the risk of chronic disease in adulthood: Engage in at least 30 minutes of moderate-intensity physical activity, above usual activity, at work or home on most days of the week.
    - For most people, greater health benefits can be obtained by engaging in physical activity of more vigorous intensity or longer duration.
    - To help manage body weight and prevent gradual, unhealthy body weight gain in adulthood: Engage in approximately 60 minutes of moderate- to vigorous-intensity activity on most days of the week while not exceeding caloric intake requirements.
    - To sustain weight loss in adulthood: Participate in at least 60 to 90 minutes of daily moderate-intensity physical activity while not exceeding caloric intake requirements. Some people may need to consult with a healthcare provider before participating in this level of activity.
- Ahieve physical fitness by including cardiovascular conditioning, stretching exercises for flexibility, and resistance exercises or calisthenics for muscle strength and endurance.

Maintaining a Physically Active Lifestyle   Maintaining a consistent physically active lifestyle is essential for preventing heart disease, maintaining healthy weight, and improving overall health and longevity. Many health benefits are associated with regular participation in intermittent, moderate-intensity physical activity. For physical activity to become a regular activity, it should be done for 30 minutes at a time (or more) per day (e.g., a 30-minute brisk walk, a 30-minute bicycle ride) at least 4 days per week. Physical activity can include such activities as walking briskly, biking, swimming, line dancing, and aerobics classes (or any other activities where the exertion is similar to these activities) (see Table 1.6). An individual's heart rate and/or breathing should increase, but exhausting oneself is not necessary.

> For more information regarding how much physical activity people need throughout the lifespan, please visit the following web site titled, "Physical Activity for Everyone": http://www.cdc.gov/nccdphp/dnpa/physical/everyone/recommendations/index.htm

Regular physical activity can be beneficial in reducing the incidence of chronic conditions in individuals with disabilities through the following: lowering blood pressure; controlling weight; improving cardiorespiratory and muscular function; preventing heart disease, diabetes, and colon cancer; maintaining healthy bones, muscles, and joints; preventing osteoporosis; increasing or improving strength, cardiovascular endurance, and balance; improving lung (pulmonary) function; reducing depression and anxiety; boosting the immune system; and reducing falls (Centers for Disease Control and Prevention, 2008b; Rimmer & Rubin, 1996).

> Foods are not generally unhealthy...but many diets are.

Diet, Nutrition, and Health

The term *diet* sometimes conjures up a negative notion of having fewer calories and regulating selection of foods to lose weight for medical or cosmetic reasons. In this way, *to diet* is used as a verb. Diet is also used as a noun. When used as a noun, diet means the usual food and drink of a person. When we talk about diet in this book, we are using it as a noun.

Well-balanced diets rich in fruits and vegetables, whole grains, lean meats/meat alternatives, and low-fat dairy foods are essential for promoting health and reducing the risk of heart disease, certain types of cancers, stroke, diabetes, osteoporosis, and early death (U.S. Department of Health and Human Services, 2005a). Good nutrition underlines good health. However, figuring out what good nutrition means still remains a challenge—especially for individuals with DD. Today we are bombarded by conflicting information about the "perfect diet," the "the zero-calorie fat substitutes," the food additives, and what to eat and when, but the bottom line is that everyone has to eat.

No matter how good or bad our food and drink choices are, those choices become our diet. Diet is one of the hardest and most challenging behaviors to change, especially since the effects of the foods eaten today may not influence a person's immediate health. One can have poor nutritional habits for years before physical or clinical symptoms occur. For example, individuals can consume a diet high in saturated fat for a very long time but eventually, as cho-

> *One can have poor nutritional habits for years before physical or clinical symptoms occur.*

lesterol deposits build up in the blood vessels, they may notice shortness of breath during physical activity. Fatty material builds up in the coronary arteries and can lead to a heart attack.

Nutrition for People with Disabilities

Nutrition can be a protective factor. Conversely, nutrition may be a risk factor for health conditions, and poor nutrition in the form of deficiencies can be a health condition itself and lead to malnutrition. Malnutrition can be described as *overnutrition* (i.e., consumption of nutrients in a pattern that leads to the development of such diseases as cardiovascular disease, cancer, or diabetes) and *undernutrition* (i.e., nutrient deficiencies leading to such conditions as anemia, osteoporosis, or wasting in adults) (Wardlaw, Insel, & Seyler, 1994). Malnutrition is a risk factor for several health issues ranging from weight problems (e.g., obesity, underweight) to dental/oral hygiene problems, bowel and bladder problems, fatigue, physical fitness/conditioning problems, diabetes, osteoporosis, and cancer. Many health conditions can further modify one's diet and create subsequent nutritional problems. For adults with DD living in a variety of settings, concerns related to food choices consist of the following: 1) nutrition knowledge is often insufficient, 2) food preparation skills are limited, 3) diets are high in fat and calories, 4) consumption of fruits and vegetables is low, and 5) limited income leads to poor food choices.

For people with disabilities, nutrient requirements should be evaluated relative to differences in activity levels, altered metabolic processes, long-term medication use, and varied modes of eating. Although our knowledge of nutrition issues for people with DD is limited, a small but growing body of research suggests that current diets are not sufficient in respect to individual nutrient and energy needs. In studies of adults with DD residing in community settings, 93% had a high-fat diet and 63%–69% did not consume enough fruits and vegetables

(Draheim, Williams et al., 2002; Sisirak et al., 2007; Sisirak, Marks, Riley, & Heller, 2008).

People with various disabilities may have specific growth, nutrient, and energy needs due to slower or faster rates of metabolism, issues with chewing and swallowing, varied modes of eating (e.g., soft diet), and lack of clarity regarding daily requirements for vitamins and minerals. For example, people with Down syndrome have caloric needs that are lower than those of their peers (on average they burn 200–300 calories less per day) (Medlen, 2002). Instead of limiting calories, which may lead to certain nutritional, vitamin, and mineral deficiencies, it may be necessary to increase their daily activity levels. Some people with autism may be at nutritional risk due to the behaviors that they may have with food and eating. Food refusal and difficulty in introducing new foods into the diet are common concerns for people with autism (Knivsberg, Reichelt, Holden, & Nodland, 2002; Knivsberg, Reichelt, & Nodland, 2001). For example, a person may only choose to eat specific types of food (e.g., dry, wet, certain colors or shapes). This type of behavior may put them at nutritional risk, especially if they omit entire food groups (e.g., vegetables or dairy). People with Prader-Willi syndrome may have soft tooth enamel; thick, sticky saliva; poor oral hygiene; and a tendency toward teeth grinding (Holm et al., 1993; Lucas & Byler, 2003). With Alzheimer's disease (AD), people may experience periods of agitation and pacing, which may lead to weight loss. Also, pathological changes in the hypothalamus affecting the regulation of food intake and metabolic processes have been observed in people who have AD (McDaniel, Hunt, Hackes, & Pope, 2001; Miziniak, 1994; Ryan, Kline, Hamrick, & Edwards, 1995).

Furthermore, individuals with DD often experience inadequate and/or irregular dental care, causing dental caries and increased risk of dental or periodontal disease, and potentially compromising nutritional status (Palmer, 2001). Due to poor dental care, tooth replacement (dental prosthesis) is common and dentures often do not fit well, resulting in difficulties with eating, chewing, and swallowing; weight loss; anorexia; and malnutrition. For more information, visit the National Center on Physical Activity and Disability (http://www.ncpad.org/nutrition).

With the high percentage of individuals taking psychotropic medications (see Table 1.7), along with a wide variety of other medications, individuals often have side effects that alter their sense of taste, texture, and smell and inhibit saliva production. Saliva is critical in that it limits bacteria, strengthens teeth, lubricates tissues, and enhances taste sensation (Palmer, 2001). Having a dry mouth may cause increases in burning/soreness, chewing difficulty, swallowing, and oral infections; and it may have an impact on food selection and dietary choices. In addition, food can affect medication absorption and metabolism, resulting in diminished nutritional status. Food/nutrients may also decrease a drug's efficacy or increase its toxicity, affecting the medication's absorption and availability, metabolism, and excretion. The presence of food in the stomach may decrease the rate and/or extent of drug absorption. For example, the effects of antihistamines may be decreased when taken with specific food such as grapefruit (Dresser, Kim, & Bailey, 2005), a high-fiber diet may decrease absorption of antidepressants (Stewart, 1992), and a high-protein diet promotes increased renal excretion of certain drugs (Welling, 1996).

Table 1.7.   Medication use among participants in a health promotion study

Medication	Participants (%)
Gastrointestinal drugs	78
Psychotropic medications	50
Hormones	38
Cardiovascular drugs (e.g., Antihypertensive, Antihyperlipidemic)	36
Respiratory drugs	33
Anticonvulsants	30
Antibacterial drugs	12
Decongestants	12
Oral contraceptives	11

# of participants (n = 190), # of drugs (n = 272).
Source: Sisirak, Marks, Riley, & Chang (2008).

For people with DD, medications can decrease or increase appetite (e.g., some anti-depressants and most "antipsychotic" drugs, such as Elavil and Mellaril), cause nausea and vomiting, and alter taste and smell (e.g., Tri-cyclic antidepressants such as amitriptyline cause dry mouth and sour/metallic taste; some antibiotics cause bitter taste).

> *For adults with DD residing in community settings, 93% have been found to have a high-fat diet, and 63%–69% of adults with DD do not consume enough fruits and vegetables.*

Where Are Meals Prepared for People with Developmental Disabilities? Information on nutrition and diets among people with DD is limited. The deinstitutionalization policies for community integration provided an opportunity for people with DD to make more choices in their daily lives. Although many people with DD still do not have the opportunity to decide where they will live or what job they will have, people with DD are increasingly living in community settings such as group homes and apartments, and they are gaining the freedom to have more responsibility for food choices. Yet, research data suggests that even in community-based housing most residents have limited involvement in food shopping (22%), meal planning (27%), and meal preparation (40%) (Sisirak et al., 2007). Furthermore, most adults with DD are eating meals that are prepared at home—breakfast (98%), lunch (94%), and dinner (100%). In regard to making food choices, 48% of people choose the food that they eat; 48% choose the food that is cooked at home, and 54% choose the portion size that they eat. People with DD also report the following related to food satisfaction: 22% of people do not think that the food they eat is healthy, and 8% are not happy with the food that they eat (Sisirak et al., 2007).

Staff, caregivers, and family members often can influence these food choices along with control over menu planning and food preparation. Caregivers report the following expected outcomes for adults with DD eating fruits and vegetables: improved overall health and cholesterol, increased ability to lose or control weight, increased energy, and reduced constipation. The following may also be barriers to improved nutrition: high staff turnover resulting in inadequate training, education, time, and experience and behavior of staff (i.e., limited staff knowledge of planning menus, buying food, and preparing foods). Additional barriers may also prevent adults with DD from eating the recommended amounts of fruits and vegetables. Top barriers to eating more fruits and vegetables reported by adults with DD in a study of staff in community-based homes included "Going bad too quickly" (60%), "Cost" (50%), "Not knowing how to prepare them" (33%), "Difficult to chew and swallow" (31%), "Take too long to prepare" (27%), "Too lazy to prepare" (22%), and "No one to show them how to prepare" (20%) (Sisirak et al., 2007).

What Is the Impact of Diet?

Food is a large part of our life and an integral part of our culture. Today, the overriding theme in nutrition research is individuality. One type of diet does not fit all and not everyone needs to be "skinny" to be healthy.

What is the impact of our diets on our lives? Each year, according to the Centers for Disease Control and Prevention (2003), more than $33 billion in medical costs and $9 billion in lost productivity due to heart disease, cancer, stroke, and diabetes are attributed to diet. Currently, few Americans have diets that meet the dietary guidelines for Americans set forth by the USDA. Americans at the beginning of the 21st century continue to expand their waistlines and consume more food and calories compared with their counterparts in the 1950s and even in the 1970s. For example, in 2000, the total annual meat consumption (red meat, poultry, and fish) reached 195 pounds per person—a 57-pound increase above the average annual consumption during the 1950s (USDA, 2003). Each American consumed an average of 7 pounds more red meat than in the 1950s, 46 lbs more poultry, and 4 lbs more fish and shellfish (USDA, 2003). In addition, people who were of normal weight ate more fruit and vegetables per day compared with their peers who were obese (Blanck et al., 2007).

What Influences Food Choices?

The primary purpose of food is nourishment, but for many people, it is more than that. Food is a large part of many social and cultural gatherings. It may be our prize—a reward—to celebrate a promotion or a good grade. It may also be our destressor and comfort. Boredom may be another factor leading people to eat more than their caloric needs. Food preferences are influenced by age, gender, cultural background, genetic makeup, occupation, and lifestyle. See Figure 1.7 for factors that determine food choices. See Figure 1.8 to consider the factors that determine your food choices.

U.S. Department of Agriculture Dietary Guidelines for Americans

New dietary guidelines for Americans were published in January 2005. They are published jointly every 5 years since 1980 by the U.S. Department of Health and Human Services (DHHS) and the USDA. The guidelines provide authoritative advice for people 2 years and older about the ways in which good dietary habits can promote health and reduce risk of acquiring major chronic diseases. They serve as the basis for federal food and nutrition education programs.

The USDA has the following key recommendations for the general population:

Consume Adequate Nutrients within Calorie Needs

- Consume a variety of nutrient-dense foods and beverages within and among the basic food groups while choosing foods that limit the intake of saturated and trans fats, cholesterol, added sugars, salt, and alcohol.

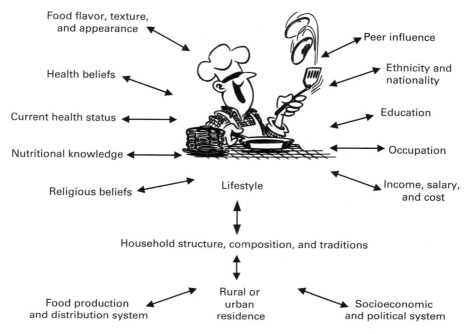

Figure 1.7. Some factors that determine food choices.

- Meet recommended intakes within energy needs by adopting a balanced eating pattern, such as the USDA Food Guide (U.S. DHHS, 2005a) or the Dietary Approaches to Stop Hypertension (DASH) Eating Plan (National Institutes of Health, 2006).

Maintain Weight by Balancing Calories

- To maintain body weight in a healthy range, balance calories from foods and beverages with calories expended.

- To prevent gradual weight gain over time, make small decreases in food and beverage calories and increase physical activity.

Visit MyPyramid.gov   In April 2005, the USDA released its completely new pyramid on its web site (http://www.MyPyramid.gov). Utilizing the newest technology, MyPyramid incorporates interactive, individualized plans and statistical tools (see Figure 1.9). Innovations of the new pyramid include quantity measures in cups instead of in serving sizes; a new symbol of physical activity (person on the stairs); an ability to track what one eats, including graphical statistics over time; and individualized recommendations to improve nutrition.

Visit MyPyramid.gov for an interactive web site that offers personalized eating plans, interactive tools to help you plan and assess your food choices, and advice that can help you and your clients to do the following:

- Make smart choices from every food group

- Find your balance between food and physical activity

		Not significant at all			Very significant	
Weight control	0	1	2	3	4	5
Health	0	1	2	3	4	5
Food costs	0	1	2	3	4	5
Convenience/Time	0	1	2	3	4	5
Family background	0	1	2	3	4	5
Advertisements (TV or radio)	0	1	2	3	4	5
Emotions	0	1	2	3	4	5
Peers (friends, co-workers)	0	1	2	3	4	5
Customs/Ethnic background	0	1	2	3	4	5
Physical activity level	0	1	2	3	4	5
Taste	0	1	2	3	4	5

INTERPRETATION

Take note of the factors that scored 4 or 5. These are your most significant influences. Next to these put a PLUS (+) or MINUS (–) sign to indicate whether you feel they have been a positive or negative influence on your health.

Figure 1.8. What factors determine your food choices? (From Wardlaw, G.M., Insel, P.M., & Seyler, M.F. [1994]. *Contemporary nutrition: Issues and insights.* Mosby: St. Louis; adapted by permission.)

- Get the most nutrition out of your calories
- Stay within your daily calorie needs

Encourage Healthy Food Choices Some tips to encourage healthy food choices include the following:

- Consume sufficient amount of fruits and vegetables while staying within caloric requirements
- Choose a variety of fruits and vegetables each day from all five vegetable subgroups (dark green, orange, legumes, starchy vegetables, and other vegetables)
- Consume three or more ounces of whole-grain products per day, with the rest of the recommended grains coming from enriched products. In general, at least half of all grains consumed should come from whole grains.
- Consume 3 cups per day of fat-free or low-fat milk or equivalent milk products.

Encouraging people to look at their eating habits is important in being able to understand why they choose the foods they do. With even small changes in attitudes toward food, chances for enjoying a long and healthy life are increased. The more people know about nutrition and their body, the better they will be able to plan and create meals that are enjoyable and that meet their needs!

Anatomy of MyPyramid

One size doesn't fit all
USDA's new MyPyramid symbolizes a personalized approach to healthy eating and physical activity. The symbol has been designed to be simple. It has been developed to remind consumers to make healthy food choices and to be active every day. The different parts of the symbol are described below.

Activity
Activity is represented by the steps and the person climbing them, as a reminder of the importance of daily physical activity.

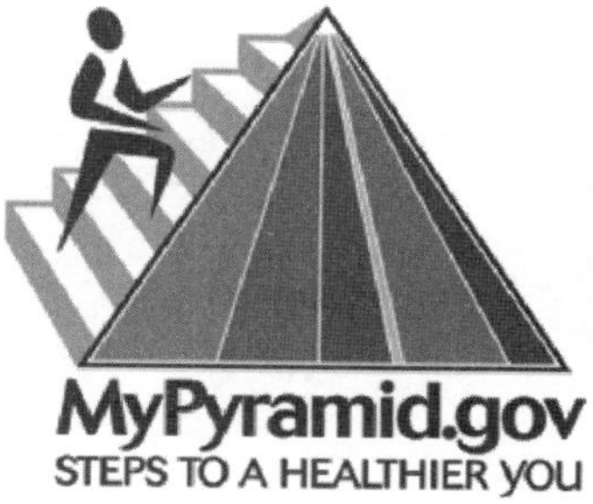

Proportionality
Proportionality is shown by the different widths of the food group bands. The widths suggest how much food a person should choose from each group. The widths are just a general guide, not exact proportions. Check the Web site for how much is right for you.

Moderation
Moderation is represented by the narrowing of each food group from bottom to top. The wider base stands for foods with little or no solid fats or added sugars. These should be selected more often. The narrower top area stands for foods containing more added sugar and solid fats. The more active you are, the more of these foods can fit into your diet.

Variety
Variety is symbolized by the 6 color bands representing the 5 food groups of the Pyramid and oils. This illustrates that foods from all groups are needed each day for good health.

MyPyramid.gov
STEPS TO A HEALTHIER YOU

Personalization
Personalization is shown by the person on the steps, the slogan, and the URL. Find the kinds of amounts of food to eat each day at MyPyramid.gov.

Gradual Improvement
Gradual improvement is encouraged by the slogan. It suggests that individuals can benefit from taking small steps to improve their diet and lifestyle each day.

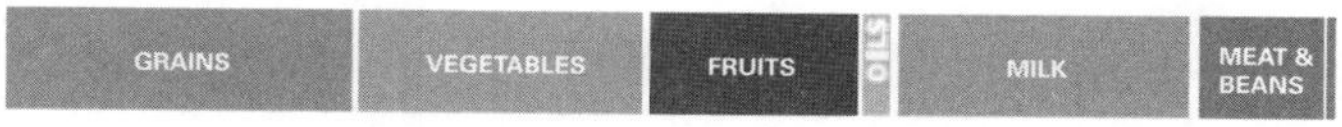

GRAINS | VEGETABLES | FRUITS | OILS | MILK | MEAT & BEANS

Figure 1.9. Anatomy of MyPyramid. (From U.S. Department of Agriculture Center for Nutrition Poliicy and Promotion (2005). *Anatomy of MyPyramid*. Retrieved January 2, 2010, from http://www.mypyramid.gov/downloads/MyPyramid_Anatomy.pdf.)

Understanding Portion Sizes The portion size (or serving size) of food affects energy intake in men and women who are of a normal weight as well as those who are overweight. Estimating serving sizes is challenging for everyone. Research has shown that people will frequently eat more if larger portions are available. For example, Rolls (2002) and her colleagues gave 51 people four different portion sizes of macaroni and cheese on different days. The bigger the portion size, they found, the more people ate—about 30% more calories when given the largest portion compared with the smallest portion.

Understanding serving sizes, along with making good food choices, is a part of healthy eating. However, visualizing a portion size can be difficult. Not knowing how much food has been consumed may result in eating hundreds of extra calories and gaining weight. Although it's difficult to estimate food serving sizes, Figure 1.10 shows some ways to help estimate serving sizes in the major food groups.

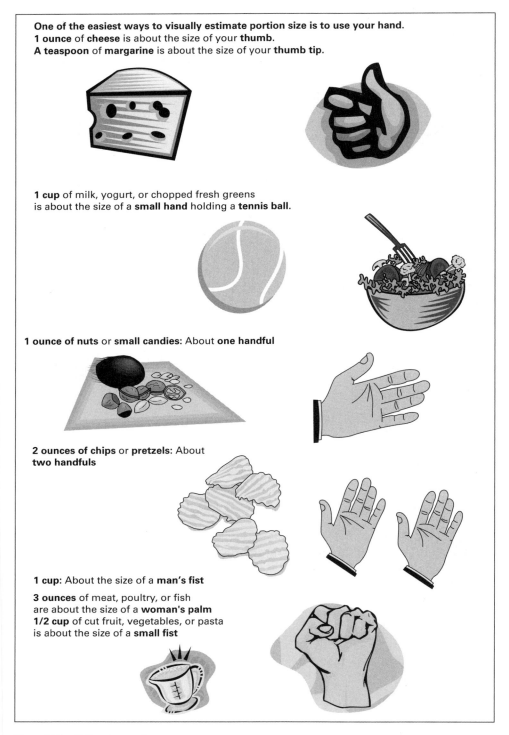

One of the easiest ways to visually estimate portion size is to use your hand.
1 ounce of **cheese** is about the size of your **thumb.**
A teaspoon of **margarine** is about the size of your **thumb tip.**

1 cup of milk, yogurt, or chopped fresh greens
is about the size of a **small hand** holding a **tennis ball.**

1 ounce of nuts or **small candies:** About **one handful**

2 ounces of chips or **pretzels:** About
two handfuls

1 cup: About the size of a **man's fist**

3 ounces of meat, poultry, or fish
are about the size of a **woman's palm**
1/2 cup of cut fruit, vegetables, or pasta
is about the size of a **small fist**

Figure 1.10.   Estimating portion sizes.

Summary

This chapter has provided an overview of factors contributing to health and wellness for adults with DD. Developing a comprehensive health promotion program requires an understanding of how lifestyle and behavior affect health for people with DD. For individuals with DD and their supports, increasing understanding of ways that exercise and nutrition influence health and of ways to promote more positive lifestyle behaviors is critical to improving their health status and participation in community life.

Behaviors
and Environment

In this chapter, we will examine the relationship between health status and health behaviors of individuals with DD within the context of their environment and culture in which they live, work, and recreate.

Factors related to behavior change—such as knowledge, attitudes, and beliefs toward physical activity and eating healthy foods—are discussed. Helpful steps to encourage individuals with DD to change their health behaviors are reviewed. Steps for starting a health promotion program within an organization are also provided. Finally, individual assessment tools and program evaluation strategies for both participants and organizations are provided.

> While a large number of individuals who are in bad health end up with a disability, a large number of persons with disabilities end up with bad health.
> — J. Rimmer (personal communication, November 17, 2009)

Factors Related to Behavior Change

Successful health promotion programs include comprehensive, targeted activities that recognize both individual and organizational factors related to behavior change. Many models continue to focus only on motivating individuals to change their behaviors. Unfortunately, many people will return to unhealthy behaviors because their environment does not recognize the influence and importance of supportive attitudes, organizational policies, and "corporate cultures" on individual behavior change.

In developing a health promotion program for people with DD, considering the relationship of an individual with a disability, his or her family and support professionals, the organizational culture of a service-related program (including work/day program and residential supports), and the environmental issues and community resources is critical. All of these factors are interconnected. Figure 2.1 depicts an ecological approach to these factors. When looking at designing, implementing, and evaluating a health promotion program, it is important to think of multiple levels of influence on behavior (McLeroy, Bibeau, Steckler, & Glanz, 1988). Behaviors are dynamic interactions between the individual and his or her

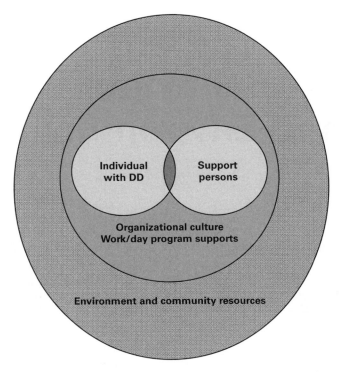

Figure 2.1.   Ecological approach to factors influencing health behavior.

environment. Factors such as knowledge, attitudes, and skills are intrapersonal, individual-based, and often have been the focal point of health education activities. Interpersonal processes and primary groups are the second level of influence on behaviors, which provide social identity, supports, and role definition. A third level of influence on individual behavior includes institutional factors such as rules and policies that are used to guide behavior of members within organizations. Community factors such as relationships among other organizations within geopolitical borders are the fourth level of influence. The final level of influence includes policy-related factors on local, state, and national levels. Incorporating a multilevel approach by including all five levels of influence on behavior will ensure greater success for your health promotion program.

Although the initiation of behavior change often starts at the individual level, developing successful health promotion programs requires taking into account multiple domains of influence—be it support persons, peers, organizational culture, media, community, and the broader society—and their impacts on an individual and his or her behavior. An ecological approach recognizes that the individual is strongly influenced by these domains, societal systems, and cultural norms. Incorporating strategies that measure, assess, and include multilevel factors will increase the success of the comprehensive health promotion program. This approach also recognizes that no one individual can change health behavior and that change needs to take place across multiple levels to truly have an impact on organizational behavior change. Using this comprehensive model allows organizations and individuals to identify and assess where they can begin to put their efforts given their strengths, resources, and experience.

Environment and Community

By recognizing the importance of environments on supporting healthy lifestyles, individuals will be better able not only to change their health behaviors but also to maintain their newly adopted health habits. *Environment* is a physically external factor that affects a person's behavior directly and indirectly (Baranowski, Perry, & Parcel, 2002). Environmental factors, such as economy, cultural and religious practices, geographic location, and media advertising influence availability, accessibility, acceptability, appropriateness, and cost of health promotion services (Conner & Armitage, 2002). For example, according to research studies, food availability in the grocery stores, cost, preparation time, and storage space limitations were identified as barriers to fresh foods in the general population (Nestle et al., 1998; Shankar & Klassen, 2001). Fruit and vegetable consumption tends to be higher when grocery stores carry more fresh produce, workplace cafeterias offer more choices at lower prices, and more healthful choices are placed in vending machines (Nestle et al., 1998).

For people with DD, readily available sources of health information may not be accurate. Television is one of the major and probably most widely used sources of health information, second only to health professionals (Nestle et al., 1998; O'Malley, Kerner, & Johnson, 1999). In the United States, watching television is one of the major sedentary activities that children and adults engage in during their leisure time (Hu, Li, Colditz, Willett, & Manson, 2003). People who watch television are exposed to a constant stream of food marketing and advertisements that have been shown to increase food and caloric intake and promote poor dietary habits (Hu et al., 2003; Wallace, 2005). Adults with disabilities tend to watch more television than the general population due to lower levels of employment and high barriers to alternative community-based leisure time activities (Bowe, 2006; Frey et al., 2005). In addition, media messages have been found to confuse people with DD on information related to health and food choice (Rodgers, 1998).

Environment can be a barrier and can also be a source of external support for a community-based organization (CBO). Being aware of community resources available in your local community can increase the success of the health promotion program. Universities and community colleges can be a wonderful resource for students to develop and implement health promotion programs within your organization. Local hospitals and clinics may also provide resources related to health fairs for health education and health risk screenings (e.g., blood pressure, cholesterol, osteoporosis, diabetes). The political climate of your community and state should also be considered in relation to funding issues and programs related to health and health promotion.

Organizational Culture

Over the past several decades, private corporations and industries have realized the impact of organizational culture on employee health behaviors and productivity (Glasgow & Terborg, 1988; Mullen, 1988; O'Donnell & Ainsworth, 1984; Schein, 1990; Warner, Wickizer, Wolfe, Schildroth, & Samuelson, 1988; Winett, King, & Altmann, 1989). Companies can identify organizational factors that support people in changing their health behaviors so that they can have healthier lifestyles. For example, organizational factors, such as programs and services, policies and procedures, and facilities and equipment, have an impact on whether or not people adopt and maintain healthy behaviors (Fielding, 1990; Glasgow, McCaul, & Fisher, 1993; Glasgow & Terborg, 1988; Mullen, 1988; O'Donnell & Ainsworth, 1984; Schein, 1999; Warner et al., 1988; Winett et al., 1989). Nonprofit CBOs that support people with DD in residential and day programs are now beginning to consider the impact of organizational factors on healthy lifestyles for people with DD receiving services and employees. For people with DD, constraints regarding group living, service structures, unclear policy guidelines, and resource limitations may predetermine and limit the availability of health promotion programming, leisure time that fosters physical activities, and the availability of healthy food options (Harris et al., 2003; Messent, Cooke, & Long, 1999).

Sustainable, comprehensive health promotion programs for people with DD require a supportive environment and attitudes within your organization. A *supportive environment* refers to the policies and procedures relating to health and safety and the provision of support for engaging in healthy behaviors. Supportive attitudes are also necessary to promote healthy lifestyles for both staff and individuals with DD.

Starting a Health Promotion Program within an Organization

The following sections detail instructions for developing a health promotion program within an organization. Some important steps to starting a health promotion program include getting support from key stakeholders and lenders, creating selling points, and recruiting others to join your health promotion program. A case scenario with follow-up questions is also included.

Getting Support from Key Stakeholders and Leaders

Gaining an understanding of senior management's expectations and motivations for starting a health promotion program within the organization is an important place to begin in getting support. Making time to meet with key leaders or the decision makers is a useful strategy in getting support to develop a health promotion program for people with DD (U.S. Coast Guard, 2001).

When initiating discussion of a health promotion program, it is good to begin by creating a core group of early adopters. Make a list of stakeholders that you will need to have "on board" in order to make a successful launch of the program. Some examples of the stakeholders are people with DD, executive director, board member, parent, staff that are highly interested in health promotion, and so forth. Start small with a few interested co-workers, and get them excited about creating an environment of health and wellness. Many organizations will have some early adopters who are interested in promoting health and who want to learn more about it and try out new ideas with their clients. Early adopter employees can serve as a core group who are able to sustain interest and enthusiasm and who work through the inevitable glitches and setbacks that occur in the early stages of a new program.

To prepare for meeting with key stakeholders and leaders, pull together materials aimed at educating management and key leaders on health promotion initiatives. The following information may be helpful in meeting with key leaders:

1. Prepare written and verbal information.

2. Use presentation materials and equipment.

3. Identify the purpose of the health promotion program.

4. Highlight the benefits of the proposed program plan.

5. Take a fact sheet or short articles about the health promotion program for key leaders to read.

6. Prepare examples and alternative plans for the key leaders to consider.

7. Talk to other organizations in your area about possible ideas and program/resource sharing.

After the meeting with management and key leaders, write a brief summary of the meeting for management to review.

Creating Selling Points

Organizations are often hesitant to spend money on health promotion programs, especially when there are other competing priorities. You may need to compete with other programs for internal funds, and show management or key leaders that using funds for your program has many benefits, including health benefits for individuals with DD and economical benefits such as lower health insurance premiums, fewer visits to the emergency room, fewer acute-care office visits, fewer and shorter hospital stays, and so forth. Health promotion programs are also an investment in the health of all people; and, controlling health care costs through the health promotion program is one of the least expensive and potentially most beneficial economic strategies.

As you start developing your program plans, it's important to remember that health promotion programs don't have to be expensive.

> *Health promotion programs don't have to be expensive.*

Consider incorporating volunteers in the program and use of low cost or free materials. For Internet resources on free materials and ideas, see Chapter 5 or visit Rehabilitation Research and Training Center on Aging with Developmental Disabilities at http://www.rrtcadd.org.

Additional points to consider include the following:

1. *Do your homework.* Work out a spending plan. For a sample budget plan, see Chapter 3.

2. *Be selective.* Choose your expenditure items carefully. For example, if you're buying exercise equipment, consider factors related to the number of people using the equipment, maintenance costs, repair costs, and equipment warranties (i.e., if you purchased "home equipment" but you are using it in a day program, your warranty may be voided).

3. *Start modestly.* Do not ask for everything the first year. Consider items that are less costly and require less maintenance (e.g., floor mats, exercise bands and balls).

4. *Show results.* Keep tabs on expenses and outcomes. Be able to show improvements. Let your participants be your spokespersons.

5. *Involve others.* The wellness committee and others can support your plan. Be open to feedback throughout the process. Make adjustments as needed.

6. *Consider timing.* Present your expense plan at the right time of the year or quarter. Do not propose a new expense plan at the end of the fiscal year when the budget is low. Be aware when the funding is starting and prepare your budget accordingly.

Recruiting Others

To gain support for starting a health promotion program, you may find it useful to identify co-workers and clients within the organization who are interested in participating in the program. Initial steps include the following:

1. Identify the most influential person in the organization who will champion and coordinate the program.

2. Discuss the proposed program with co-workers and clients/residents.

3. Explore strategies that will support a new health promotion program that incorporates physical activity and health education classes. For example, for your "core group," you may consider individual abilities and qualities, such as the ability to model positive health behaviors, the ability to work well with individuals with DD and their support persons, and the ability to provide an influential role in the decision-making process. To get additional support, you may consider recruiting volunteers from a variety of places. First, if your agency has a volunteer pool, talk to volunteers who have an interest in health promotion activities. Your board members may also be a source of support. Students enrolled in schools for health professionals (i.e., adapted physical education, nursing, nutrition, health education, exercise physiology, physical therapy, occupational therapy, recreational therapy) may also be interested to volunteer with community agencies to fulfill coursework requirements.

CASE SCENARIO

Weight Complaints

The management team in a community-based organization providing housing for adults with DD has been receiving many complaints from parents about the tremendous weight gain among their sons and daughters who are living in group homes. Parents are requesting that this issue be addressed immediately throughout all areas in the organization.

Q1: What plan should the management team develop to address this issue?

Q2: What barriers might be expected in implementing this plan?

Q3: What are some potential resources that the management team can use to ensure the success of the proposed plan?

Understanding the Transtheoretical Model of Change for Your Health Promotion Program

Motivating people to change their behavior can be viewed as a continuum related to a person's readiness to change. *Change*, in this case, is an event occurring over time. Readiness to change can be identified by using the five stages of the Transtheoretical Model of Change (TTM). TTM is a theoretical model of behavior change developed in the 1980s and is still being used extensively as the basis for developing effective interventions to promote health behavior change (Prochaska & DiClemente, 1983; Prochaska, DiClemente, & Norcross, 1992; Prochaska et al., 1994). The TTM is a model of intentional change focusing on the decision making of the individual. The model has previously been applied to a wide variety of topics, such as smoking cessation, exercise, low-fat diet, radon testing, alcohol abuse, weight control, organizational change, use of sunscreens to prevent skin cancer, drug abuse, medical compliance, mammography screening, and stress management. The five stages in the TTM consist of Precontemplation, Contemplation, Preparation, Action, and Maintenance (Prochaska & DiClemente, 1992).

Precontemplation Stage

- No intention to make changes

- Denial of a specific health or health-related problem

- Blaming external factors

In the Precontemplation Stage, an individual is often unaware or underaware of the need to change their behavior. You may focus your activities on increasing the individual's understanding of health, physical activity, and nutrition, along with making decisions about his or her health, by giving the individual more information and resources. For example, if a person has never understood why fiber would be of benefit to him or her, he or she most likely would not perceive the benefits of eating more fresh fruits and vegetables or whole grain products (foods high in fiber) for better health. By giving a person more information and teaching him or her the benefits of fiber (e.g., fiber reduces the risk of colon cancer, fiber makes your digestion regular), you are making that individual think about whether he or she should make a change.

Contemplation Stage

- Considering a change

- Identifying advantages/disadvantages

- Focusing on internal factors

As a person moves into the Contemplation Stage, he or she has the necessary information and knowledge, is becoming aware of the need to change his or her behavior, and is seriously thinking about change. In the Contemplation Stage, however, a person has not yet made a commitment to take action. Essentially, a person in this stage understands the benefits of changing a particular behavior (e.g., eating more fiber), but he or she is still looking at the positive and negative benefits of making a change. In this stage, a person will consider lifestyle change and assess his or her behaviors.

Preparation Stage

- Deciding to change

- Making small changes and significant changes

People are ready to take action and change a specific behavior in the Preparation Stage. At this Stage, a person will focus on setting goals and examining barriers and influences that may affect his or her ability to exercise or eat a more nutritious diet. For example, a person may think about specific topics related to starting a health promotion program, such as having enough money to join a gym to exercise regularly. Or, if he or she wants to increase his or her fresh fruit and vegetable intake, he or she may start identifying the stores that may have good produce, the distance to the stores from home, and the cost of the fresh fruits and vegetables.

Action Stage

- Setting goals

- Developing an action plan

- Seeking support

- Monitoring progress

- Obtaining rewards

In the Action Stage, a person is taking action and has changed his or her health behavior(s). For example, a person may now be exercising and trying to include healthy foods in his or her diet. The primary focus in this stage is on reinforcing new behaviors to maintain exercise and nutrition goals. For example, a person has made his or her goal to exercise three times a day and eat five servings of fresh fruits and vegetables. The person has identified different exercises that he or she wants to do and has planned his or her meals incorporating fresh fruits and vegetables.

Maintenance Stage

- Sustaining the change over time

- Using coping skills

- Monitoring progress

- Seeking support

A person is considering ways to prevent relapse (stopping the new health-promoting behavior) when he or she is in the Maintenance Stage. Activities are focused on reviewing what an individual has learned and different ways to continue with his or her program. During this phase, a person may need support in developing coping strategies to use when there are changes in his or her daily routines, such as holidays and vacations. Supporting an individual to identify appropriate rewards is an important component in being successful in maintaining behavior change.

At any time during the five stages of change, people may stop their health promoting behavior. In working with people with DD, you may find it easier to state this as a period of "getting off track" instead of using the TTM term of *relapse*. Holiday time is the most common time when people get out of their usual food and exercise regimens. This is why gym memberships increase in the month of January: People usually make a New Year's resolution to get back on track.

Rates of Behavior Change

It is believed that many people go through the five stages of behavior change at different rates. In fact, people often move back and forth between stages a number of times before they maintain their behavior change goals. Figure 2.2 shows how behavior change is cyclical rather than a linear process. In general, people use different processes (or activities) to move from one stage of change to another, so it's important to target the right activity (process) at the right time (stage).

In using this model, you can tailor your activities to match a person's stage of readiness to change his or her behavior. For example, for someone who is not

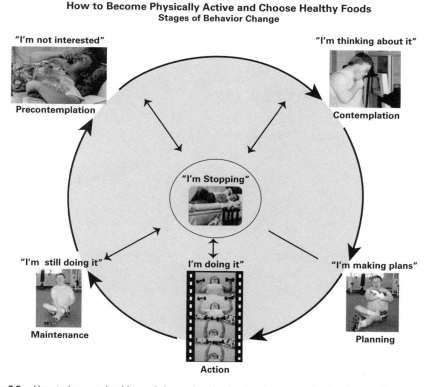

How to Become Physically Active and Choose Healthy Foods
Stages of Behavior Change

"I'm not interested"
Precontemplation

"I'm thinking about it"
Contemplation

"I'm Stopping"

"I'm still doing it"
Maintenance

I'm doing it"
Action

"I'm making plans"
Planning

Figure 2.2. How to become healthy and choose healthy foods: Stages of behavior change. (From Marks, B., Sisirak, J., & Heller, T. [2010]. *Health matters: The exercise and nutrition health education curriculum for people with developmental disabilities* [p. xiv]. Baltimore: Paul H. Brookes Publishing Co.; reprinted by permission.)

interested in becoming more active, you may find that encouraging a step-by-step movement along the continuum of change may be better than encouraging that person to move directly into action.

As a practice tool to see what stage you are in for doing regular physical activity, use a questionnaire such as the one in Figure 2.3. You can use this tool to think about participants whom you are supporting to determine their stage of physical activity and how to best target health education messages. You can use a similar practice tool for stages of change on eating more fruits and vegetables (see Figure 2.4).

REGULAR PHYSICAL ACTIVITY: For physical activity to be regular, it must be done for *30 minutes at a time* (or more) per day, and be done *at least* 4 days per week. For example, you could take a 30-minute brisk walk or ride a bicycle for 30 minutes. Physical activity includes such activities as walking briskly, biking, swimming, line dancing, and aerobics classes or any other activities where the exertion is similar to these activities. Your heart rate and/or breathing should increase, but there is no need to exhaust yourself.

Please answer all questions with either Yes or No.

According to the definition above:

1. Do you currently engage in regular physical activity?   ○ Yes   ○ No

2. Do you intend to engage in regular physical activity in the next 6 months?   ○ Yes   ○ No

3. Do you intend to engage in regular physical activity in the next 30 days?   ○ Yes   ○ No

4. Have you been regularly physically active for the past six months?   ○ Yes   ○ No

SCORING

If item 1 = NO and item 2 = NO	Precontemplation
If item 1 = NO and item 2 = YES and item 3 = NO	Contemplation
If item 1 = NO and item 3 = YES	Preparation
If item 1 = YES and item 4 = NO	Action
If item 1 = YES and item 4 = YES	Maintenance

Figure 2.3. What stage are you in for physical activity? (From Nigg, C., Hellsten, L., Norman, G., Braun, L., Breger, R., Burbank, P., et al. [2005]. Physical activity staging distribution: Establishing a heuristic using multiple studies. *Annals of Behavioral Medicine, 29*[2], 35–45; reprinted by permission.)

REGULAR INTAKE OF FRUITS AND VEGETABLES: Recommended intake of fruits and vegetables is 5 to 9 servings per day. For example, one serving equals one medium apple or orange, four broccoli florets, four large lettuce leafs, or anything that can fit in the palm of your hand.

Circle the answers below that best represent your fruit and vegetable intake and intentions.

How many servings of fruits and vegetables do you usually eat each day?

| 0 Zero 1 One 2 Two 3 Three 4 Four | 5 Five to nine |

Do you intend to start eating 5 or more servings of fruits and vegetables a day in the next 6 months?

1. No, and I do NOT intend to in the next 6 months.

2. Yes, I intend to in the next 6 months.

3. Yes, I intend to in the next 30 days.

Have you been eating 5 or more servings of fruits and vegetables a day for less or more than 6 months?

4. Less than 6 months.

5. More than 6 months.

SCORING

If you circled 0 to 4 servings and circled item # 1	**Precontemplation**
If you circled 0 to 4 servings and circled item # 2	**Contemplation**
If you circled 0 to 4 servings and circled item # 3	**Preparation**
If you circled 5 to 9 servings and circled item # 4	**Action**
If you circled 5 to 9 servings and circled item # 5	**Maintenance**

Figure 2.4. What stage are you in for fruit and vegetable intake? (From Laforge, R.G., Greene, G.W., & Prochaska, J.O. [1994]. Psycho-social factors influencing low fruit and vegetable consumption. *Journal of Behavioral Medicine, 17,* 361–374; adapted by permission.)

Using the Transtheoretical Model for Organizational Change

Although research examining the TTM for changing organizational behavior is limited, increased consideration is being given to TTM to examine organizational readiness. Individual motivation, combined with organizational and environmental support, tend to lead to behavior change. That is to say, within an organization, employees' behaviors are the heart of organizational change (Prochaska, 2001). Specifically, a singular focus on motivating individuals to change their behaviors is not enough. If an environment does not value the importance of attitudes among

> *Individual motivation, combined with organizational and environmental support, tend to lead to healthy behavior change.*

workers, policies, and the overall work culture of an individual's behavior, people may return to their unhealthy behaviors. In addition, research across a range of behaviors and populations suggests that only 20% of individuals are currently in the Preparation Stage (Laforge, Velicer, Richmond, & Owen, 1999; Prochaska, Prochaska, & Levesque, 2001; Velicer et al., 1995). People may be resistant to take any kind of new action if they are not in the Preparation Stage. Studies have documented that if a high number of employees are in the Preparation Stage, an organization-wide intervention will be successful (Prochaska et al., 2001). Administrators in CBOs and researchers need to understand what stage the majority of people within an organization are in order to utilize the appropriate processes to guide people, both individuals with DD and any employees, through the stages of behavior change.

Using Assessments in Your Health Promotion Program

Understanding employees' knowledge, attitudes, and skills related to health promotion activities provides useful information to develop organizational health promotion goals, objectives, and strategies. People are better able to maintain healthy behaviors when their environment recognizes the influence and importance of attitudes, organizational policy, and "corporate cultures" on individual behavior change. Assessing knowledge, attitudes, and skills about physical activity and nutrition for people with DD among CBOs is a useful way to develop and integrate health promoting activities throughout all areas of service.

As you begin to think about starting a health promotion initiative, we have found it useful to have a timeline (see Figure 2.5) that details the items that need to be completed. In addition, having an understanding of the amount of effort required

> *Assessing knowledge, attitudes, and skills about physical activity and nutrition for people with DD among CBOs is a useful way to develop and integrate health promoting activities throughout all areas of service.*

to plan, develop, implement, and evaluate a health promotion program (see Figure 2.6), along with the various components of your organizational and health promotion program plan (refer to Figure 2.7), can assist you in moving your program from ideas to action to sustainability. Note the numbers 2–5 in boxes in Figures 2.5 (left side), 2.6 (bottom), and 2.7 (bottom). They correspond to the Chapter numbers and will be discussed in more detail in the subsequent chapters.

Types of Assessment

The first step in developing a sustainable health promotion program is to become familiar with the health needs and health-related interests of your clients,

Activity	Month	1	2	3	4	5	6	7	8	9	10	11	12
2	Convene program planning group.	▓											
	Review organizational policies for health promotion and share with stakeholders.	▓											
	Conduct employee and organizational needs and asset assessments.	▓											
3	Translate assessment information into action plan and objectives and share with stakeholders.		▓										
	Integrate *Health Matters* curriculum into existing staff training *(optional)*.				▓	▓	▓	▓	▓	▓	▓		
	Integrate *Health Matters* curriculum into new hire training *(optional)*.				▓	▓	▓	▓	▓				
	Advertise for program personnel.			▓	▓								
	Hire and train program coordinator.					▓	▓						
	Advertise the health promotion program to stakeholders.					▓	▓						
	Train program personnel (staff).						▓	▓					
	Conduct baseline evaluation: Get doctor's consent, psychosocial survey, and fitness test for adults with developmental disabilities (DD).							▓	▓				
4	Deliver the health promotion program.									▓	▓	▓	▓
5	Conduct postproject evaluation: Conduct psychosocial survey and fitness test for adults with DD.											▓	
	Collect staff and participant feedback about program.							▓	▓				
	Conduct process evaluation.		▓	▓	▓	▓	▓	▓	▓	▓	▓		
	Analyze evaluation data.											▓	
	Produce report.												▓
	Disseminate report (internally and externally).												▓
	Conduct future directions planning.												▓

*Marks, B., Sisirak, J., & Heller, T. (2010). *Health matters: The exercise and nutrition health education curriculum for people with developmental disabilities.* Baltimore: Paul H. Brookes Publishing Co.

Figure 2.5.   Sample timeline for Year 1 development of a health promotion program. (From Issel, M.L. [2004]. *Health program planning and evaluation: A practical, systematic approach for community health* [p. 214]. Sudbury, MA: Jones & Bartlett Publishers; adapted by permission.)

employees, and organization. Also, considering the resources that are available in your community is critical. This process may entail a variety of assessments. Four general types of assessments include 1) an organizational needs assessment, 2) an organizational capacity assessment, 3) a marketing assessment, and 4) a community health assessment (Issel, 2004). Each of these assessments are discussed briefly in the following sections.

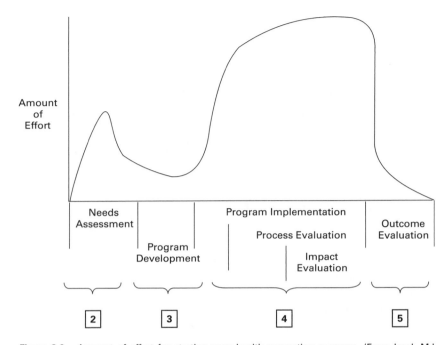

Figure 2.6. Amount of effort for starting your health promotion program. (From Issel, M.L. [2004]. *Health program planning and evaluation: A practical, systematic approach for community health* [p. 214]. Sudbury, MA: Jones & Bartlett Publishers; adapted by permission.)

Needs Assessment for Your Organization

As mentioned, Figure 2.6 highlights the importance of dedicating time to conduct a needs assessment prior to any type of program development for health promotion. Assessing needs within your organization consists of identifying the types of health promotion programs and services that are available for clients and employees and the accessibility of facilities and resources for staff and clients/residents to be physically active and make healthy food choices. Please refer to the Appendix: Health Matters Assessments, for the assessment form.

A needs assessment should simultaneously be done among potential participants with DD to prioritize health-related issues (e.g., overall health status, obesity rates, pain, depression, fitness levels, knowledge of exercise and healthy food choices, engaging in physical activity and making healthy food choices). Assessing individual factors may include the following health status components: physical, psychological, and social.

In assessing physical measures, you may consider assessing baseline measures (measures taken before you start a program) of heart rate, blood pressure, body composition measurements of height and weight to calculate body mass index, and waist and hip circumference (to calculate waist-hip ratio as a measure of body fat). Depending on your program, you may want to assess measures of flexibility, aerobic capacity, balance, and strength of upper and lower body muscles (FABS). Specific tests for each component of FABS may consist of the following:

- **Flexibility:** Behind the Back (upper body flexibility) and Sit and Reach (lower body flexibility)

- **Aerobic/Cardiovascular Capacity:** 6-Minute Walk Test

**Diagram of the Components of the Organizational Plan and
Health Promotion Program Plan**

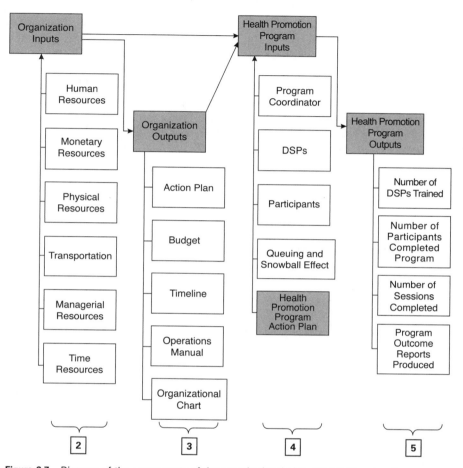

Figure 2.7. Diagram of the components of the organizational plan and health promotion program plan. (From Issel, M.L. [2004]. *Health program planning and evaluation: A practical, systematic approach for community health.* Sudbury, MA: Jones & Bartlett Publishers [p. 215]; adapted by permission.)

- **Balance:** Timed Get-Up-and-Go (TGUG) Test

- **Strength and Endurance:** YMCA Bench Press (upper body strength) or One-Minute Timed Sit-to-Stand Muscular Endurance Test (lower body strength)

You may also consider assessing psychosocial measures related to the following: exercise and nutrition knowledge, social and environmental support for exercise and making healthy food choices, and attitudes (pros and cons of exercise and eating fruits and vegetables); and confidence (perceived self-efficacy) to exercise regularly and eat fruits and vegetables. For a detailed Testing Procedure Manual on how to conduct physical and psychosocial tests, along with the specific scales, please refer to *Health Matters: The Exercise and Nutrition Health Education Curriculum for People with Developmental Disabilities* (Marks et al., 2010). (See Figure 2.8 for an example of the Fitness Data Collection Form from the Testing Procedure Manual.)

Fitness Data Collection Form

Participant's name: _____   ID number: _____

Interviewer's name: _____   ID number: _____

Date: _____

Test period (circle response):

Pretest (T1)   Posttest (T2)   6-month posttest (T3)   1-year posttest (T4)

Heart Rate, Blood Pressure, and Cholesterol Measurements

Heart rate: _____   Blood pressure: _____

Currently on high blood pressure medication?   Yes   No   Don't know

Currently on cholesterol lowering medication?   Yes   No   Don't know

Cholesterol results

   Total cholesterol (TC): _____

   Triglycerides: _____

   High density lipoprotein (HDL): "Good" cholesterol: _____

   Low density lipoprotein (LDL): "Bad" cholesterol: _____

   TC/HDL ratio (risk of heart disease): _____

Figure 2.8.   Example of a Fitness Data Collection Form from the Testing Procedure Manual.

From Marks, B., Sisirak, J., & Heller, T. (2010). *Health matters: The exercise and nutrition health education curriculum for people with developmental disabilities* (p. 379–381). Baltimore: Paul H. Brookes Publishing Co; reprinted by permission. Copyright © 2010 by Paul H. Brookes Publishing Co. All rights reserved.

In *Health Matters for People with Developmental Disabilities: Creating a Sustainable Health Promotion Program*, by Beth Marks, Jasmina Sisirak, & Tamar Heller (2010, Paul H. Brookes Publishing Co.)

Figure 2.8. *(continued)*

Fitness Data Collection Form

Body Composition Measurements

Height, Weight, and Waist-to-Hip Circumference

Measurement   Circumference

Height: _____ _____ _____   Waist:_____ _____ _____

Weight: _____ _____ _____   Hip: _____ _____ _____

Body Mass Index (BMI): _____   Blood pressure: _____

Flexibility Measurements

Shoulder Flexibility Test

Left side   Right side

_____ cm   _____ cm

_____ cm   _____ cm

_____ cm   _____ cm

Sit-and-Reach

Shoes (circle one):   On   Off

_____ inches

_____ inches

_____ inches

Aerobic/Cardiovascular Fitness Measurements

Six-Minute Walk Test

Lap tally (cross lap number after each lap):

1	2	3	4	5	6	7	8	9	10
11	12	13	14	15	16	17	18	19	20
21	22	23	24	25	26	27	28	29	30

Total number of laps = _____

End time (indicate if not exactly 6 minutes): _____ minutes

Calculate total number of yards = _____

Number of laps x 50 yards + extra yards (if less than a full lap of 50 yards, to the closest 5-yard segment)

(continued)

Figure 2.8. *(continued)*

Fitness Data Collection Form

Balance Measurements

Timed Get-Up-and-Go Test

_____ seconds   _____ seconds   _____ seconds

Strength and Endurance Measurements

**One-Minute Timed
Modified Pushup Test**   Number of pushups: _____

YMCA Bench Press Test   Number of repetitions: _____

**One-Minute Timed Sit-to-Stand
Muscular Endurance Test**   Number of repetitions: _____

One-Repetition Maximum (1-RM) Test   Maximum weight: _____ lbs

Equipment: _____   Maximum weight: _____ lbs

Equipment: _____   Maximum weight: _____ lbs

Equipment: _____   Maximum weight: _____ lbs

Equipment: _____   Maximum weight: _____ lbs

Assessment of Organizational Capacity

Changing individual behaviors must be considered within the context of where people live, work, and recreate. Conducting an organizational assessment is a critical step in understanding the capacity—that is, Strengths, Weaknesses, Opportunities, and Threats (SWOT)—within the organization in developing, providing, and sustaining a comprehensive health promotion program for individuals with disabilities. Organizational factors to consider may consist of internal resources, organizational culture, employee knowledge related to health promotion, and employee skills and attitudes related to health promotion activities. Figure 2.7 can be used as a guide for understanding the factors to consider within your organization to support your health promotion program. Organizational inputs may include human, monetary, and physical resources; transportation options; and managerial and time resources.

Organizational outputs can include an action plan, budget, timeline, operations manual, and organizational chart reflecting health promotion activities. As you identify your organizational inputs and outputs, you can then begin formalizing your inputs for the health promotion program, which consists of identifying interested participants and staff and creating a "snowball effect." In other words, you want to create momentum by having a group to initiate the program and a "waitlist" of people who will be in the second and third health promotion program groups. Once you have started your health promotion program, it's important to begin to assess the program outputs. This can include items such as number of staff (or support persons) trained, number of participants who completed the program, number of sessions completed, and reports generated.

Marketing Assessment

Although you always want to identify health needs and concerns among your target audience, you also want to consider the interest level of your key participants. Ensuring that both people with disabilities and support persons are interested in participating in a new health promotion program is necessary for longterm sustainability. A marketing assessment seeks to answer the question, "What will motivate the target audience to join the program?" This assessment process will help you identify other competing programs and available resources in the community.

Community Health Assessment

A community health assessment will give you a better profile of major health issues and the magnitude of the identified health problem in your community or neighborhood. This process can help you understand the priority that your community gives to a particular health issue. Also, you can gain insight into the available health and human services resources and assets, as well as community weaknesses. For example, does your local community have an infrastructure that has an indoor community facility for physical activity and exercise that is affordable and accessible for community residents with disabilities? If there is an indoor recreational facility, does it include aerobic exercise equipment, such as stationary cycles or stairmasters that are accessible for people with disabilities? Is there strength-training equipment that is accessible? Do employees at the recreational facility feel comfortable working with people who have DD and have the capacity to instruct people on using the machines? Does your local community have accessible outdoor recreation and walking trails?

Within your local community, do restaurants serve healthy food alternatives, fresh fruits or vegetables, or healthy beverage alternatives? Do fast-food restaurants provide labels (e.g., low-fat, light, heart healthy) to identify healthy food alternatives, or do they label foods on the basis of nutritional value (e.g., calories, fat grams, percent of calories from fat)? Do local grocery stores have good quality fruits (dried or fresh), low-fat snacks, or other healthy food alternatives that are affordable? Do the vending machines provide labels that identify healthy food alternatives on or near the vending machines? Do the labels indicate nutritional value provided on or near the vending machines (e.g., fat grams, percent of calories from fat)?

Health Matters Assessments

The Health Matters Assessments (Marks, Sisirak, & Donahue-Chase, 2008) found in the Appendix can be used to assess your organization's health promotion needs and capacity for supporting a health promotion initiative within the context of your local community. The Health Matters Assessment of Needs (HMAN) and Health Matters Assessment of Capacity (HMAC) can be used in developing new programs based on organizational and individual needs, interests, and resources that will support clients/residents with DD and/or employees in engaging in healthy behaviors. In addition, the HMAC can be used to evaluate your health promotion program on multiple levels, including individual capacity, employee capacity, organizational resources, and community resources.

The HMAN (Marks, Sisirak, & Donahue-Chase, 2008) was developed to assess the types of health promotion programs and services available for clients and employees within an organization. The HMAN also assesses the types of promotional messages for healthy behaviors or health promotion programs. Does your organization provide healthy eating or physical activity messages to clients or employees through posters, newsletters, or brochures? Measures assessing the level of support for physical activity and healthy food choice within an organization's environment are also included. For example, does your organization assist in accessing facilities that enable staff and clients/residents to be physically active or making healthy food choices? See Appendix A for assessment tools.

Culture change within an organization requires a comprehensive, systematized and continuous revision of cultural influences, such as training, available resources, rewards, and communication strategies. A complex and sustained cultural shift within an organization requires the development and implementation of a strategic plan for a creating a supportive health-promoting environment. The HMAC (Marks, Sisirak, & Donahue-Chase, 2008) was developed to assess perceptions of knowledge, skills, resources, and commitment of employees across all levels of the organization. See the Appendix for these tools within the HMAC.

Use of the HMAC can assist management in CBOs to develop and implement health promotion programs for people with DD and the CBO employees. In addition, the HMAC was developed for management to conduct internal and external benchmarking within their organization and across similar types of CBOs. The HMAC tool can be used to develop strategic plans related to health promotion goals and objectives aimed at creating a culture of health and wellness throughout the organization. The spidergram in Figure 2.9 can be used to map the priority areas on a yearly basis that need to be targeted for monies and efforts.

In general, the questions on the HMAC aim to determine employee perceptions in four general areas: 1) organizational culture (commitment, policies, and structures), 2) knowledge, 3) confidence and attitudes, and 4) resources (internal and external). Within organizational culture, do leaders, managers and staff enable and support health promotion practice and values? Is there a sense of commitment within the organization? Do employees believe in and advocate for health promotion? Do the vision, mission, and policies support health promotion activities? The HMAC also assesses an employee's perception of his or her knowledge of the fundamental principles and strategies of health promotion and his or her confidence and attitudes in being able to support persons with DD to exercise, eat healthy, and be successful in a health promotions program. Last, employees are queried as to their perceptions of having the necessary resources to implement health promotion activities.

Specific items relating to organizational culture address the value of health promotion within the organization (i.e., is information conveyed clearly; do job descriptions and performance reviews include health promotion activities). In essence, did everyone "Get the Memo" about health promotion in the organization?

An employee is also asked about his or her perceived knowledge and confidence level in being able to provide health promotion to people with DD (i.e., does employee know health risk factors; does employee understand the importance of health promotion and health promotion strategies; does employee include personal preferences in health promotion activities with his or her client;

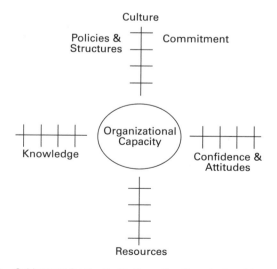

Figure 2.9. Spidergram for the Health Promotion Organizational Assessment

does employee believe that he or she can teach information related to nutrition or exercise).

The HMAC includes items for employees' perceptions regarding organizational and community resources for health promotion activities (i.e., is there adequate time, equipment/resources, support from manager and co-workers, to do health promotion activities; are fitness-related supplies, cooking utensils, and/or recipes readily available; are health promotion trainings and programs provided to people with DD and employees; do employees and people with DD have access to financial and community resources for activities).

Last, a demographics section is also provided to determine areas within the organization that may need specific types of support. For example, employees in a day program may have different needs related to resources or policies and procedures compared with employees in a residential program. You may also see differences in employees across job descriptions. Direct support staff often struggle with adequate resources, but feel very confident in working with individuals with DD. Or, you may find that new employees have different training needs (i.e., less confidence in teaching, less knowledge about specific types of disabilities related to health promotion) than do employees who have been in the job longer.

Evaluating Physical Health Status   The physical health status assessment measures general health; body composition; height, weight, and waist-to-hip circumference; flexibility, aerobic, balance, and strength abilities; and psychosocial well-being and health. Staff who support people with DD also can be queried regarding client's health status, energy levels, functional status, medications, history of falls, adherence to healthy behaviors, physical activity levels, health conditions, and health care utilization.

Physiological health can be evaluated by measuring blood pressure, body composition, and waist circumference. Physiological health can also be evaluated by assessing flexibility, aerobic capacity, balance, and strength.

Blood Pressure   Blood pressure is measured using standardized criteria (Reeves et al., 1995). After the person has been seated for 5 minutes, blood pressure is measured with the appropriate size blood pressure cuff or an electronic wrist blood pressure cuff. The average of two consecutive blood pressure measurements should be used. Measurements should be taken from the individual's left arm.

Body Composition   Height, weight, and waist and hip circumference can be taken on each participant by trained personnel. Body Mass Index (BMI) is a measure of body fat relative to height and weight, whereas waist circumference measures abdominal fat. Combining these two measures with information on risk factors for diseases and conditions associated with obesity can yield one's risk for developing obesity-associated diseases.

BMI is a person's weight in kilograms divided by the square of his or her height in meters, or a person's weight in pounds divided by the square of height in inches times 703. Too much body fat can be a problem because it can result in illnesses and other health problems. National Heart, Lung, and Blood Institute (NHLBI, 1995) has the following guidelines for BMI: < 18.5, underweight; 18.5–24.9, normal; 25.0–29.9, overweight; 30–39.9, obese; and 40+, extremely obese. BMI can be calculated using the following formula:

$$\text{BMI} = \left(\frac{\text{Weight in Pounds}}{(\text{Height in inches}) \times (\text{Height in inches})} \right) \times 703$$

The BMI measure has limitations in that it can overestimate body fat in athletes and others who have a muscular build and underestimate body fat in older adults and others who have lost muscle mass. For example, two people can have the same BMI, but they can have a different percent of body fat. A bodybuilder with a large muscle mass and a low percent body fat may have the same BMI as a person who has more body fat because BMI is calculated using weight and height only.

Waist Circumference Measuring waist circumference is another good indicator of abdominal fat and another predictor of your risk for developing heart disease and other diseases. This risk increases with a waist measurement of more than 40 inches in men and more than 35 inches in women. Another factor to consider in assessing overweight status includes additional health risk factors for diseases and conditions associated with obesity. These risk factors include the following: blood pressure (hypertension), high LDL-cholesterol ("bad" cholesterol), low HDL-cholesterol ("good" cholesterol), high triglycerides, high blood sugar (glucose), family history of premature heart disease, physical inactivity, and cigarette smoking.

Flexibility Lower leg and back flexibility can be measured using the Sit-and-Reach Test for the lower extremities. Test–retest reliability for the Sit-and-Reach test ranges from $r = .93$ to $r = .97$ (American College of Sports Medicine; 2006; Heyward, 2006; Hui & Yuen, 2000). Upper body flexibility can be measured using the Shoulder Flexibility Test (Miotto, Chodzko-Zajko, Reich, & Supler, 1999; Rikli & Jones, 1999).

Aerobic Capacity The 6-Minute Walk Test (6-MWT) has been validated and is a simple, safe, and low-cost field test that is used to assess cardiopulmonary fitness and functional exercise capacity (American Thoracic Society, 2002; Enright, 2003; Kervio, Carre, & Ville, 2003; Oh-Park, Zohman, & Abrahams, 1997; O'Keefe, Lye, Donnellan, & Carmichael, 1998). The 6-MWT can be used in older adults as well as in younger individuals. A significant correlation has been obtained between VO2max and Anthrometric values and 6-MWT parameters ($r = 0.97$, (r^2) = 0.94, $p < 0.01$) with at least two familiarization tests.

Balance The Timed Get-Up-and-Go (TGUG) Test (Podsiadlo & Richardson, 1991; Wall, Bell, Campbell, & Davis, 2000) is another simple, safe, and low-cost field test that is used to assess a person's gait and balance (agility and coordination). It is a useful functional measure to assess an individual's risk of falls by having a person stand (from a sitting position) without using their arms for support, walk 10 feet, turn and return to the chair, and sit back in the chair without using their arms for support.

Strength and Endurance for Upper and Lower Body Muscles Upper body muscular strength and endurance can be measured with a handgrip dynamometer or using the YMCA Modified Bench Press (YMCA of the USA, 2000). Lower body muscle strength and endurance can be evaluated using the One-Minute Timed Sit-to-Stand Muscular Endurance Test, which measures muscle strength and endurance of large leg muscles by counting the number or correct sit to stands executed during a 1-minute period (Bohannon, 1995; Gross, Stevenson, Charette, Pyka, & Marcus, 1998).

Evaluating Psychosocial Health Status Many tests can be used to evaluate psychosocial health outcomes for your health promotion program, including a single-item question to evaluate general health status (Ware & Sherbourne, 1992), energy/fatigue (Ware & Sherbourne, 1992), functional status (Lorig et al., 1996), current medications, history of falls, and health care utilization. Several scales that you may consider using include the Child Depression Inventory Scale (CDI-S) adapted for adults (Ailey, 1996; Kovacs, 1985) to evaluate psychosocial well-being, the Life Satisfaction Scale (Heller, Sterns, Sutton, & Factor, 1996), the Pain Scale (Granger et al., 1994), and Choice-Making Inventory (Heller, Miller, Hsieh, & Sterns, 2000) are discussed in the next sections.

Energy/Fatigue The level of energy and fatigue can be assessed using Energy/Fatigue Scale (Ware & Sherbourne, 1992). This is a verbal rating scale of fatigue intensity. It consists of six questions with a five-choice response format containing adjectives describing both fatigue (worn out, tired) and energy (pep, energy).

Functional Status Functional Status Scale (Lorig et al., 1996) measures whether the participant's health interferes with their social roles and activities.

Psychosocial Well-Being Depression can be assessed with the Child Depression Inventory Scale (CDI-S) (Kovacs, 1985), which was adapted for adults with DD. In the adapted version, the alpha reliability is .79 and test–retest reliability is 60 (Ailey, 1996). CDI-S is a copyrighted scale and can be purchased. However, the Glasgow Depression Inventory is available free of charge and has two versions, one for people with intellectual disabilities and one for caregivers.

Life Satisfaction Scale Life satisfaction can be assessed using the Life Satisfaction Scale, which was developed specifically for adults with intellectual disabilities. It has been demonstrated to have good alpha reliability (alpha = .81 to .82) and test–retest reliability (.60 to .83). Its domains include satisfaction with health, leisure/recreation, work, residence, and social support. It is administered through interviewing participants (Hawkings, Ardovino, & Hsieh, 1998; Heller et al., 1996; Lawton, Moss, Fulcomer, & Kleban, 1982).

Pain The level of pain can be assessed using the Pain Scale, which has been validated with older participants living in community settings (Granger et al., 1994). The Pain Scale consists of seven items that ask questions about the pain when performing activities of daily living (e.g., walking, climbing stairs, getting in and out of a chair, putting clothes on).

Choice-Making Inventory The amount of independence and autonomy that people with DD have when making their choices is measured with the Choice-Making Inventory (Heller, Miller, et al., 2000). It has demonstrated good consistency (alpha = .85).

Evaluating Physical Activity and Nutrition Knowledge and Supports Evaluations that can be used to measure physical activity and nutrition knowledge and supports include measures of attitudes and beliefs about exercise (Heller et al., 2004; Heller & Pochaska, 2001), barriers to exercise (Heller et al., 2004; Heller, Rimmer, & Rubin, 2001), the Self-Efficacy (Confidence) to

Exercise (Heller et al., 2004; Heller, 2001a; Lorig et al., 1989), social and environmental supports for exercise (Heller, 2001b), attitudes, beliefs, and barriers to eating fruits and vegetables (Sisirak et al., 2007; Sisirak et al., 2008), social and environmental supports to nutrition (Sallis, Grossman, Patterson, Pinski, & Nader, 1987) and the Nutrition and Activity Knowledge Scale (Illingworth, Moore, & McGillivray, 2003).

Attitudes and Beliefs About Exercise Perceived outcomes are measured by the Exercise Perceptions Scale (Heller & Pochaska, 2001), which includes nine items assessing the perceived benefits of exercise for oneself (self-rating) or for the person with DD. This instrument is rated on a Likert scale from 1 (*strongly disagree*) to 5 (*strongly agree*) for the informant and from 1 to 3 for the person with a disability. The alpha reliability is .79, and test–retest is .72.

Barriers to Exercise Items in the Barriers to Exercise Scale (Heller, Rimmer, et al., 2001) include respondent's perception toward participating in physical activity in community settings or alone, knowledge of exercise, exercise accessibility, preferences, and respondent's reasons for not being involved in exercise. The Barriers to Exercise Scale includes 18 items about barriers toward exercise participation, including motivation, knowledge, accessibility, and social barriers. Both participants and informants are asked identical questions. It is rated on a 3-point-Likert scale from 1 (*not a barrier*) to 3 (*yes, a barrier*) for the person with DD and a 5-point-Likert scale from 1 (*strongly disagree*) to 5 (*strongly agree*) for the informant. When comparing the two scales, the informant's scale is recoded into a 3-point rating. The overall reliability is .73, and test–retest reliability is .55.

Self-Efficacy (Confidence) to Exercise The Self-Efficacy to Perform Exercise instrument includes five items pertaining to the confidence that one has in performing exercises for muscle strength and flexibility and in performing aerobic exercises (Heller et al., 2004).

Social/Environmental Supports Scale This scale examines who provides support to facilitate exercise, including family, friends, health professional, or service provider staff. This is a 6-item scale with alpha reliability of .76 and test–retest reliability of .48 (Heller et al., 2001b).

Attitudes and Beliefs about Eating Fruits and Vegetables Perceived outcomes of eating fruits and vegetables are measured by the Fruit and Vegetable Perceptions Scale (Sisirak et al, 2008; Sisirak et al., 2007), which includes 7 items for staff/caregivers and 10 items for people with DD assessing the perceived benefits of eating fruits and vegetables. This measure is rated on a Likert scale from 1 (I disagree very much) to 5 (I agree very much) for staff/caregivers and from 1 to 3 for people with DD.

Barriers to Eating Fruits and Vegetables Scale includes 15 items for staff/caregivers and 13 items for people with DD. This measure is rated on a Likert scale from 1 (strongly disagree) to 5 (strongly agree) for staff/caregivers and from 1 to 3 for people with DD.

Barriers to Eating Fruits and Vegetables Items in the Barriers to Eating Fruits and Vegetables Scale (Sisirak et al., 2008; Sisirak, et al., 2007) include respondent perception toward fruit and vegetable cost, cooking, time, ability to chew and swallow, and perceived health benefits.

Social/Environmental Supports for Nutrition   The four items examine who provides support to people with DD to eat healthier food options, including family, friends, health professionals, or service provider staff (Sallis et al., 1987).

Nutrition and Activity Knowledge Scale (NAKS)   Nutrition and Activity Knowledge Scale (NAKS; Illingworth et al., 2003) is an 18-item, picture-based scale designed to assist with the assessment of nutrition and activity knowledge and was developed specifically for adults with DD to assess nutrition and activity knowledge. The scale focuses on assessing knowledge as it relates to weight gain and loss and the energy needs of people participating in different activities. The illustrations are designed to assist in ensuring that the question is understood by the respondent. Cronbach's alpha is satisfactory for both factors: α = .71 (weight/weight control) and α = .59 (nutritional value of food) and for the total scale α = .78. Test-retest reliability for the weight/weight control subscale was r = .83 (p<0.001), r = .69 (p<0.001) for the nutritional value of food subscale, and r = .82 (p<0.001) for the total scale (Sisirak, Marks, & Heller, 2005). Please contact the authors for more information about this scale.

Evaluating Adherence to Healthy Behaviors   Evaluating adherence to healthy behaviors includes activity level in a typical day and the type of activities that are being done (CDC, n.d.; Lorig et al., 1996; Sallis et al., 1987); nutrition, including servings of fruits and vegetables per day; amount of water an individual drinks; smoking habits; and alcohol use.

Evaluating Your Health Promotion Program

Evaluation is a critical component to build into health promotion programs. By having a thorough evaluation plan you will be able to continually improve, adapt, and adjust your existing program to meet the needs of participants and your organization. Different types of evaluations will help you to understand how your health promotion program works, give feedback to your participants, improve your program, and describe your program so that it can be replicated. Program evaluation consists of collecting information about various aspects of a program, such as the following: cost/benefit analysis,

> *Evaluations can help your participants, improve your program, and describe your program so that it can be replicated.*

effectiveness, efficiency, and process and outcome evaluation. Evaluating your health promotion program can allow you to do the following (McNamara, 2008):

1. *Understand, verify, or increase the impact of services and programs for people with DD and employees.* These outcome evaluations are increasingly required by nonprofit funding bodies to verify that their monies are helping their constituents. Service providers can understand what their customers or clients need and provide unbiased reports on how the new services could be delivered.

2. *Improve delivery mechanisms to be more efficient and less costly.* Without program evaluation, service delivery may end up being an ineffective collection of activities that are less efficient and more costly than needed. Evaluations can identify program strengths and weaknesses to improve the program and adapt and adjust it to meet the needs of people with DD and your organization.

3. *Verify that you're doing what you think you're doing.* Typically, plans about how to deliver programs and services end up changing substantially as those plans are put into place. Evaluations can verify if the program is really running as originally planned.

4. *Facilitate management.* This way management is really thinking about the goals of their program, what their program is all about, and how their program is able to meet their goals.

5. *Produce data or verify results.* The data can be used to understand how your program helps participants, gives feedback to participants and staff in the program, improves public relations, and promotes your services in the community.

6. *Generate valid comparisons.* Generating valid comparisons between programs can help decide which programs should be retained in the face of pending budget cuts.

7. *Examine effective programs.* Fully examine and describe effective programs for replication in other CBOs.

Questions for Evaluating an Exercise and Health Education Program

A general program evaluation can be completed by employees in CBOs who provide day and residential programs for people with DD. For example, the HMAN can be done on an annual basis to document improvements related to health promotion activities, ongoing gaps, and emerging issues. When completing a general program evaluation, there are several aspects to keep in mind, such as the purpose of the evaluation and the kind of evaluation that is necessary for your program.

What is your purpose? Consider the following questions:

1. Why are you doing the evaluation (i.e., what do you want to be able to decide as a result of the evaluation)?

2. Who will be receiving the results of the evaluation (e.g., participants with disabilities, funding organizations, board, management, staff)?

3. What kind of information do you need to either make necessary decisions and/or enlighten your intended audiences (e.g., strengths and weaknesses of the program, benefits to people with DD, how and why the program failed)?

4. What are the sources of information or who will provide feedback (e.g., participants with disabilities, staff, parents, management)?

5. How can that information be collected (e.g., using questionnaires, conducting interviews, examining documentation, observing people with DD or staff, conducting focus groups among people with DD or staff)?

6. Who will manage the data? (Data management is one of the critical steps that is often overlooked. Identifying an internal or external data management person/organization is imperative in producing final reports and analyses. A data manager should have some basic skills in statistics to run frequencies and compare before-and-after program results. Make sure that you have a budget line for data management.)

7. When do you need the information (e.g., when are quarterly/final reports due to your funding body; is there a fiscal report that your organization publishes each year)?

8. What resources are available to collect the information (e.g., make sure your staff is trained to collect the data and that the time it takes to collect the data has been budgeted. Refer to the Appendix.)?

What type of evaluation do you want to do? Consider the following types of evaluations:

1. Goals-based evaluations (Is your program meeting your objectives?)

2. Process-based evaluations (Do you understand your program's strengths and weaknesses?)

3. Outcomes-based evaluations (Can you identify benefits to participants?)

Note: It's good to do a mixture of all three types of evaluation.

Goals-Based Evaluations

Goals-based evaluations identify the extent to which your program is meeting pre-determined goals or objectives. Here are some questions to ask yourself when designing an evaluation to see if you reached your goals:

- Were the health promotion program goals and objectives effective?

- What is the status of the program's progress toward achieving the goals?

- Will the health promotion program goals be achieved according to the timelines specified in your program plan? If not, then why?

- Do personnel have adequate resources (e.g., money, equipment, facilities, training) to achieve the goals?

- Should priorities be changed to put more focus on achieving the goals?

- Should timelines be changed?

- Should goals be changed, added, or removed? If so, why?

- How should goals be established in the future?

Process-Based Evaluations

Process-based evaluations are aimed at understanding how your health promotion program works. In other words, how does your program produce results? Process-based evaluations are particularly useful in both identifying problems and potential solutions. Some questions to consider in a process evaluation include the following:

- What is required to implement your health promotion program?
- How are staff trained?
- How do participants start the program?
- What is required of participants?
- What is required of staff?
- How do staff decide what services to provide?
- What do participants and/or staff think are program strengths?
- How is staff being trained to run the program?
- What complaints do participants and/or staff have?
- What suggestions do participants and/or staff have to improve the program?
- Have you been able to get participants and staff interested in your program?
- Have you presented it to management and received support?

Outcome-Based Evaluations

Program evaluations that focus on outcomes are becoming increasingly important for nonprofit organizations. In particular, outcomes-based evaluations focus on identifying the benefits of your program to participants. Outcomes-based evaluations can help answer whether your program is really doing the right activities to bring about the outcomes you need (rather than just engaging in busy activities). What are the benefits of your health promotion program to people with DD? For example, is there an enhanced learning or change in attitudes of participants? Is there an improved physical activity adherence? Are participants eating more nutritious foods? Are participants encountering improved psychosocial and physiological health (McNamara, 2008)? Outcomes-based evaluations would provide answers to these types of questions.

Specifically, it is important to consider whether participants have the following outcomes after completing the health promotion program: 1) improved psychosocial health, 2) improved physiological health, 3) improved physical activity and nutrition knowledge and supports, and 4) improved adherence to physical activity and to eating nutritious foods.

In the previous sections, we have provided a brief overview of each of the common assessments for the four different types of participant outcome measures. The Testing Procedure Manual and Health Matters Assessments should be used as baseline data to assess client needs across the organization and as a measure of program success. Please refer to the Appendix for Health Matters Assessments. The Testing Procedure Manual can be found in *Health Matters: The Exercise and Nutrition Health Education Curriculum for People with Developmental Disabilities* (Marks, Sisirak, & Heller, 2010, Paul H. Brookes Publishing Co.). (See Figure 2.8 for an example of the Fitness Data Collection Form from the Testing Procedure Manual.)

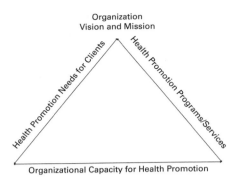

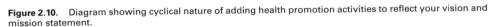

Figure 2.10. Diagram showing cyclical nature of adding health promotion activities to reflect your vision and mission statement.

The diagram in Figure 2.10 depicts the cyclical nature of adding health promotion activities to reflect your vision and mission statement within your strategic plan. As you identify needs within your organization and among your clients and understand your capacity for supporting programs and services, you can begin to identify goals for your organization and for persons with DD.

Summary

This chapter examined the relationship between individuals with DD's health status and health behaviors within the context of their environment and culture in which they live, work, and recreate. Factors related to behavior change, such as knowledge, attitudes, and beliefs toward physical activity and eating healthy foods were discussed. Steps for initiating and implementing a health promotion program within an organization were provided. Finally, individual assessment tools and program evaluation strategies for both participants and organizations were provided.

3

Setting Goals with Individuals and Your Organization

This chapter identifies strategies for setting realistic goals that support individuals with DD to change their health behaviors. Tools are provided to develop organization goals that support healthy lifestyles for people with DD and their support persons within organizations. Strategies for developing mutual goals with individuals with DD for changing health behaviors are identified. We also present a checklist and sample budget for designing a program plan to implement a physical activity and health education program.

In thinking about developing goals, it is critical to include individuals with disabilities as well as your employees. Many programs start out with a focus on individuals with disabilities. For a program to be sustainable, however, we have found that expanding the focus to organizational goals is useful in creating an infrastructure that will support long-term lifestyle changes. Goal planning is your opportunity to develop your "written map" of individual and organizational outputs. Refer back to Chapter 2, Figure 2.7, to review the essential organizational outputs including the following: 1) action plan, 2) budget, 3) timeline, 4) operations manual, and 5) organizational chart. Remember, this is your development phase (see Figure 2.6), and you should set a solid foundation before you implement your new health promotion program. Please review activities in Figure 2.5 that will help guide you as you start thinking of your next steps.

The next section contains a case study for you to think about as you read this chapter.

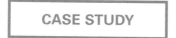

CASE STUDY

Rights and Responsibilities

The management team in your agency does not want to implement a new program for healthy food alternatives (e.g., vending machines) because they believe that this would infringe on the rights of people with DD by restricting their choices. Many staff, however, believe that the new program could teach their clients about healthier food alternatives that could, in turn, improve their health.

Q1:   *What plan should staff develop to address this issue?*

Q2:   *What barriers might be expected in implementing this plan?*

Q3:   *What are some potential resources that the management team can use to ensure the success of the proposed plan?*

Developing Organizational and Participant Goals

Developing a sustainable, comprehensive health promotion program for people with DD requires a supportive environment and supportive attitudes within your organization. A *supportive environment* refers to the policies and procedures relating to health and safety and level of support for healthy lifestyle behavior. *Supportive attitudes* are related to the staff and management views toward healthy lifestyle for people with DD and for themselves.

We have found that people frequently want to immediately develop programs focused on changing behaviors among people with DD. Although such programs can be effective in the short term, you may want to consider three different levels of program goals (United States Coast Guard, 2001). These levels consist of the following:

1. *Awareness*: Goals are aimed at management, staff, and people with DD becoming aware of how lifestyle affects well-being for both themselves and individuals with DD.

2. *Education*: Goals are directed at management, staff, and people with DD participating in structured learning programs to prepare for behavior change. Management provides support for health promotion activities.

3. *Behavior change*: Goals are aimed at management, staff, and people with DD developing and implementing programs that support behavior change.

It is important to consider these levels of program goals when promoting activities within your organization. In other words, begin building an infrastructure supporting healthy lifestyles before starting a targeted health promotion program for people with DD.

Table 3.1 details three levels of program activities and their corresponding program goals that can be considered as you begin to develop your programs. This table also includes examples of activities that can be done to meet the goals for the three types of activities. If your goal is directed at awareness of the impact of healthy lifestyles for individuals with disabilities, you may start by including information about health and wellness in your organization's newsletter.

As noted in Table 3.1, educational goals can be achieved by creating a wellness committee that includes all stakeholders (e.g., people with disabilities, support staff, management, volunteers, family members, board members, community representatives). Some organizations have also initiated health promotion programs through an annual health fair or health screening. Health fairs are a useful strategy for providing experiential learning in that people are taught about the impact of health behaviors and gain insights into their own health habits. For example,

Table 3.1. Types of program activities, program goals, and sample activities

Program activities	Goal	Examples
Awareness	Provide educational information on the benefits of healthy lifestyle.	Handouts Posters and information posted on bulletin boards Pamphlets Fact sheets Flyers
Education	Create an environment promoting health lifestyles through policies, activities, and physical and staff resources.	Wellness committee Health fairs and screenings Fitness testing Contests Workout policies Equipment training Volunteers
Behavior change	Develop health promotion programs supporting healthy lifestyles.	Physical fitness classes Health education classes on making healthy food choices Contests and incentive-based activities

Adapted from U.S. Coast Guard. (2001) *Designing your program workbook*. Available at http://www.uscg.mil/WORKLIFE/.

people can learn about the benefits of physical activity and the problems related to high blood pressure and high cholesterol levels.

The program activities aimed at awareness and education provide a nice segue into the development of specific programs for individuals with disabilities and employee health programs. As people increase their awareness of the need for and the impact of health promotion on health, you will have a greater chance of building support among people with DD and their support staff. People will be more likely to participate in physical activity programs and health education classes if they are aware of the need for health promotion activities and understand why such activities may be beneficial. For example, as a smoker, you may be

> *Begin building an infrastructure supporting healthy lifestyles before starting a targeted health promotion program for people with DD.*

more likely to participate in a smoking cessation program if you are aware of the risks associated with smoking and have some information on various options that you can take to stop smoking.

Developing and Modifying Goals

Developing health promotion goals within your organization is an important first step before working with people with DD to establish their individual goals. Goals must be explicitly stated so that people can actually see and measure the progress in attaining the goal. If a goal cannot be measured, then it's probably not a realistic or tangible goal.

> *Goals must be explicitly stated so that people can actually see and measure the progress.*

In thinking about creating goals, it's good to imagine whether or not you can experience the goal yourself and what types of steps are necessary to meet each goal. We have found it useful to have a variety of options as people develop organization and individual goals. Initially, many people find it easier to choose a goal from several alternatives rather than trying to identify a unique goal.

Developing Organizational and Individual Goals

Organizations have a wide range of internal and external resources. We have seen organizations with very few monetary resources develop wonderful programs using limited physical resources but having their staff embrace the value of health promotion and their role in supporting healthy lifestyles for their clients. In these situations, organizations can succeed by relying on the internal abilities of each of their employees. Health promotion programs can be implemented in many types of settings, time constraints, and space restrictions. As such, it's important to have an understanding of the following issues:

1. The number of participants (people with DD) and the number of staff who are available and interested

2. The types of assistive devices and technology used by participants

3. The available time for exercise and health education classes

4. The availability of space for exercise and health education classes

5. The type of equipment available for each type of exercise

The Program Plan Inventory   The Program Plan Inventory (see Figure 3.1) can be used as a guide to determine how many people will be participating and the number of staff who will be participating in the program. In addition, the Program Plan (see Figure 3.2) can be used as a worksheet to develop program goals and objectives and a step-by-step health promotion plan. Some major questions to consider include the following:

1. *Who are the participants with DD, and how many people do you have?* The goals that you develop must consider your group size. If you are expecting participants to achieve specific psychosocial and physical health outcomes, you will need to consider having a smaller class size in order to provide the necessary staff support that is needed to ensure that individuals are able to achieve mastery over their new skills related to physical activity and nutrition.

2. *How many staff are available for the health promotion program and interested in working in teaching health education and physical activity sessions?* Do you have one to three people working for you, or do you have six or more staff? Although it's great to have many interested staff, you really want to find staff who are not only interested but also willing to experience failure along with the many successes. Despite the best-designed plans, many plans and goals must be modified. Staff should be willing to learn from things that do not work and to try new ideas. Having a few staff who work very well together can often achieve more than having many staff who do not have a close working relationship. As you design your class size, consider the impact of having a

(text continues on page 69)

Program Plan Inventory

1.   How many participants are in the program?

☐   2–5
☐   6–9
☐   10+

We have found that the ideal number is 6–8 participants per group. If you're planning to have a larger group, you may consider breaking it up in two sections for a more tailored, hands-on approach.

2.   What is the number of staff available for each session?

☐   1
☐   2–3
☐   4–5
☐   6+

A larger staff increases motivation and program intensity, and it also minimizes the risk of injury. Plan to have at least 1 staff member per 2–4 participants with disabilities. The number of staff will depend on individual needs of participants.

3.   How much time do we have available for each session?

☐   Less than 1 hour
☐   1–2 hours
☐   3 or more hours

4.   How many sessions per week can we have?

☐   1
☐   2
☐   3
☐   4 or more

5.   What is the size of the space* for the program?

☐   Average basement
☐   Average living room (17' x 23')
☐   A small gym with a basketball court (36' x 72')
☐   A regular classroom size

*Space should be free of unnecessary furniture and sharp objects that may increase the risk of falls and injury and large enough that everyone fits in comfortably.

(continued)

Figure 3.1.   Program Plan Inventory.

Figure 3.1. *(continued)*

---

6. **What kind of assistance do our participants use?**

    ☐ Braces (orthotics)/artificial limbs (prosthetics)

    ☐ Cane/crutches/walker

    ☐ Hearing device

    ☐ High-tech devices (e.g., augmentative communication, voice recognition, environmental controls)

    ☐ Low-tech devices (e.g., reacher, pen grip)

    ☐ Personal assistant

    ☐ Service animal

    ☐ Visual device

    ☐ Wheelchair (manual)

    ☐ Wheelchair (power) or scooter

    ☐ None

    ☐ Other: Please specify:_____

7. **What resources and equipment do we have available?**

    Flexibility:

    ☐ Yoga straps

    ☐ Yoga mats

    Aerobic:

    ☐ Climber/stepper

    ☐ Cross trainer

    ☐ Elliptical machine

    ☐ Exercise balls

    ☐ Exercise bike

    ☐ Jumping ropes

    ☐ Rowing machine

    ☐ Treadmill

    Balance:

    ☐ Balance board/stands

    ☐ Balance discs

    ☐ Balance domes

    ☐ Balance mats

    ☐ Exercise balls

(continued)

Figure 3.1.   *(continued)*

Strength:

- ☐ Arm machines
- ☐ Dumbells/free weights
- ☐ Fitness tubes
- ☐ Leg machines
- ☐ Medicine balls
- ☐ Resistance bands
- ☐ Exercise bands

Other:

- ☐ Blood pressure monitor
- ☐ Exercise videos
- ☐ Heart rate monitors/watches
- ☐ Mats
- ☐ Measuring wheel
- ☐ Pedometers
- ☐ Stop watch/timers
- ☐ Measuring tape

8. **Do we have staff members who are doing and/or are interested in specific health-promoting activities and/or exercises?**

   ☐ Yes   ☐ No

What activities?

- ☐ Cooking
- ☐ General exercise
- ☐ Martial arts
- ☐ Running
- ☐ Swimming
- ☐ Tai-chi
- ☐ Weight lifting
- ☐ Yoga

Program Plan

Instructions: Fill out your own program plan using the Program Plan Inventory.

1. Number of participants:

2. Number of staff available for each session:

3. Time available for each session:

4. Number of sessions per week:

5. The size of the exercise space*:

6. Assistance used by clients who will be participating in the program:

7. Equipment available:

Flexibility:

Aerobic:

Balance:

Strength:

Other:

8. Activities that staff members are doing and/or are interested in doing:

_____

*Space should be free of unnecessary furniture and sharp objects that may increase the risk of falls and injury and large enough that everyone fits in comfortably.

Figure 3.2.   Program Plan.

lower staff-to-individual with DD ratio to increase motivation, intensity, and the length of the individual program and to minimize the risk of injury. Some of the best classes that we have seen have had one staff per two to three participants with disabilities. The participant dynamics within the program are also important. If people do not get along outside of the program (e.g., if they fight), they are unlikely to become best friends in the program.

3. *How much time is available for exercise and health education classes?* Do you have less than 1 hour, 1–2 hours, or 3 or more hours? How many sessions per week can you have? Can you have two or three sessions per week lasting 1–2 hours? Or, can you only have one session per week lasting several hours? Again, the amount of time that you have will help you develop measurable and realistic program goals.

4. *How much space is available for exercise and health education classes?* Health promoting activities can be done just about anywhere. We have seen classes take place in houses, community recreation centers, day programs, work sites, churches, and schools. The important piece is to plan where you want your exercise and health education classes to occur and ensure that you will have this space for the duration of the program. Consistency helps with adherence to program goals. Just like going to school, you want your participants to know where they are going for each class. Within each space selected, you may consider two primary specifications: 1) that the space is free of unnecessary furniture and sharp objects that may increase the risk of falls and injury and 2) that the space is large enough that everyone fits in comfortably.

5. *What kind of assistance do individuals with DD who will be participating in the program use?* As you design your program goals, consider the range of assistive devices that participants use. Types of assistance may include the following: braces (orthotics) or artificial limbs (prosthetics); cane, crutches, or walker; hearing devices; high-tech devices (e.g., augmentative communication, voice recognition, environmental controls); low-tech devices (e.g., reacher, pen grip); personal assistant; service animal; visual device; wheelchair (manual or power); or scooter.

6. *What resources and equipment do you have available?* Although it is not necessary to have equipment to implement an exercise/physical activity program, you may think about whether you have equipment for each of type of exercise (e.g., flexibility, aerobics, balance, strength). For flexibility activities you may consider yoga straps or yoga mats. Aerobic exercise may incorporate a climber/stepper, cross trainer, elliptical machine, exercise balls, exercise bike, jumping ropes, rowing machine, and/or treadmill. Balance board/stands, balance discs, balance domes, balance mats, and Thera bands and balls can be used for balance exercises. A variety of equipment can be used for strength exercises including arm machines, dumbells/free weights, fitness tubes, leg machines, medicine balls, resistance bands, and Thera bands. Other useful items may include an electronic wrist blood pressure monitor, exercise videos, heart rate monitors/watches, mats, measuring wheel, pedometers, stop watch/timers, and a measuring tape.

7. *Do you have staff members who are doing and/or are interested in specific health promoting activities and/or exercises?* You can tap into your staff's

internal resources. Some staff, while not chefs, are talented cooks. You may want to ask staff members if they have experience in cooking, general exercises, martial arts, running, swimming, Tai-chi, weight lifting, and yoga, and if they would be interested in teaching some of the classes in these areas.

As you develop your organization's health promotion program plan, it's important to include the goals of your participants with DD when creating the program. Working with participants to identify the types of exercises/physical activities and nutrition activities that they want to try and finding a place in which they can do it is critical to the success of your program. Please see samples in My Goals for the Program (Figure 3.3), Participant Worksheets: Exercise Plan (Figure 3.4) and Nutrition Plan (Figure 3.5), for creating goals for participants with DD. Figure 3.3 can be used with potential participants with DD to guide you in establishing a customized health promotion program for your client. If clients have goals related to exercise and nutrition, you can use the Participant Worksheets: Exercise Plan and Nutrition Plan (see Figures 3.4 and 3.5) to identify specific strategies for achieving their goals. In addition, if clients are working on exercise goals, you may want to determine their physical activity stage using the What Stage Are You in for Physical Activity? questionnaire (see Figure 2.3 in Chapter 2). This questionnaire will provide useful information that can be used in the health education and fitness classes to develop target teaching strategies. Similarly, if clients have nutrition goals, along with the Participant Worksheet: Nutrition Plan in Figure 3.5, you can use the What Stage Are You in for Fruit and Vegetable Intake? questionnaire in Figure 2.4 in Chapter 2. Although many people may not have had experience with different types of activities and may not be able to identify a variety of activities, it is helpful to obtain baseline information as to what types of things people enjoy doing. One primary goal of the health promotion program is to give people the opportunity to experience and gain confidence in being able to engage in a variety of physical activities.

Physical Activity Readiness Questionnaire (PAR-Q)   Regular physical activity can be fun. Furthermore, increasing physical activity is very safe for most people. If you are planning a fitness program as a component of your overall health promotion strategic plan, we recommend that all participants in your program obtain approval from their health care provider before they start becoming much more physically active. All participants should complete a medical history questionnaire and a Physical Activity Readiness Questionnaire (PAR-Q; see Figure 3.6 for the first page of the 2-page form) (Canadian Society for Exercise Physiology, 2002). The PAR-Q should be completed by staff who are familiar with each person with DD.

The PAR-Q was developed to exclude people with contraindications to exercise, identify people who have an increased risk for disease, identify people with clinically significant disease, and determine the needs of each person. In general, if someone is planning to become more physically active and they are between the ages of 15 and 69, the PAR-Q is recommended as a tool to increase safety during exercise testing and participation and to assist in the development of a sound, effective exercise program.

The PAR-Q is the minimum recommended standard for screening. The PAR-Q can tell you if someone between the ages of 15 and 69 should talk with his or her health care provider before increasing their physical activity. If an individual is over 69 years of age and is not used to being very active, he or she should also check with his or her health care provider.

My Goals for the Program

Name: _____

These are some ideas of goals that you may have as you start your health education and exercise classes. As you go through the classes, you may want to add new goals or change your old goals.

1. Help me learn new things
2. Make my body feel good
3. Make me hurt less
4. Help me get in shape
5. Improve my health
6. Make my blood pressure better
7. Make me lose/control my weight
8. Help me make healthier choices
9. Make me feel less tired
10. Make me feel happier
11. Help me meet new people
12. Make me look better
13. Lower my cholesterol level
14. Improve my strength
15. Improve my balance

Goals: _____

_____

_____

_____

_____

Steps that I will take to reach my goals: _____

_____

_____

_____

_____

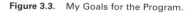

Figure 3.3. My Goals for the Program.

Exercise Plan

Name: _____

I have decided that I will spend _____ minutes per day exercising.

I would like to exercise the following days:

Monday   Tuesday   Wednesday   Thursday   Friday

Saturday   Sunday

The exercise(s) that I would like to try to do (or try) are:

_____ Exercises like we've been doing in the gym (e.g., weights, bike, rowing machine)

_____ Exercises like we've been doing in class (e.g., Yoga, Tae Bo, aerobic, dancing)

_____ Other _____

I want to do my exercises in the (use the clock to draw in the hands for the time)

_____ Morning

_____ Afternoon

_____ Evening

I want to do my exercises at

_____ Home

_____ Work

_____ Other _____

Figure 3.4.   Participant Worksheet: Exercise Plan.

Nutrition Plan

Name: _____

I have decided that I will cut down on the following foods:

I have decided that I will eat more of the following foods:

My favorite snacks (junk foods) are:

I will eat the following snacks (junk foods) (note how much per day/week)

___ Morning   _____ Home

___ Afternoon   _____ Work

___ Evening   _____ Other_____

Figure 3.5.   Participant Worksheet: Nutrition Plan.

Collecting information about age, health status, symptoms, and risk factors in the screening process is prudent. The goal is to accurately determine each person's risk of complications from exercise by answering the questions in Figure 3.6.

In general, people who are considered at low risk on the PAR-Q include younger individuals (men less than 45 years of age and women less than 55 years of age) and those who have no more than one risk factor (e.g., hypertension, obesity, hypercholesterolemia, family history). People who are considered at moderate risk on the PAR-Q include older individuals (men 45+ years of age and women 55+ years of age) or those who meet the threshold for two or more risk factors. People who are considered at high risk include individuals who have one or more

---

Physical Activity Readiness
Questionnaire - PAR-Q
(revised 2002)

PAR-Q & YOU

(A Questionnaire for People Aged 15 to 69)

Regular physical activity is fun and healthy, and increasingly more people are starting to become more active every day. Being more active is very safe for most people. However, some people should check with their doctor before they start becoming much more physically active.

If you are planning to become much more physically active than you are now, start by answering the seven questions in the box below. If you are between the ages of 15 and 69, the PAR-Q will tell you if you should check with your doctor before you start. If you are over 69 years of age, and you are not used to being very active, check with your doctor.

Common sense is your best guide when you answer these questions. Please read the questions carefully and answer each one honestly: check YES or NO.

YES	NO		
☐	☐	1.	Has your doctor ever said that you have a heart condition <u>and</u> that you should only do physical activity recommended by a doctor?
☐	☐	2.	Do you feel pain in your chest when you do physical activity?
☐	☐	3.	In the past month, have you had chest pain when you were not doing physical activity?
☐	☐	4.	Do you lose your balance because of dizziness or do you ever lose consciousness?
☐	☐	5.	Do you have a bone or joint problem (for example, back, knee or hip) that could be made worse by a change in your physical activity?
☐	☐	6.	Is your doctor currently prescribing drugs (for example, water pills) for your blood pressure or heart condition?
☐	☐	7.	Do you know of <u>any other reason</u> why you should not do physical activity?

If **you** **answered**

YES to one or more questions

Talk with your doctor by phone or in person BEFORE you start becoming much more physically active or BEFORE you have a fitness appraisal. Tell your doctor about the PAR-Q and which questions you answered YES.

- You may be able to do any activity you want — as long as you start slowly and build up gradually. Or, you may need to restrict your activities to those which are safe for you. Talk with your doctor about the kinds of activities you wish to participate in and follow his/her advice.
- Find out which community programs are safe and helpful for you.

NO to all questions

If you answered NO honestly to <u>all</u> PAR-Q questions, you can be reasonably sure that you can:
- start becoming much more physically active – begin slowly and build up gradually. This is the safest and easiest way to go.
- take part in a fitness appraisal – this is an excellent way to determine your basic fitness so that you can plan the best way for you to live actively. It is also highly recommended that you have your blood pressure evaluated. If your reading is over 144/94, talk with your doctor before you start becoming much more physically active.

DELAY BECOMING MUCH MORE ACTIVE:
- if you are not feeling well because of a temporary illness such as a cold or a fever – wait until you feel better; or
- if you are or may be pregnant – talk to your doctor before you start becoming more active.

PLEASE NOTE: If your health changes so that you then answer YES to any of the above questions, tell your fitness or health professional. Ask whether you should change your physical activity plan.

<u>Informed Use of the PAR-Q</u>: The Canadian Society for Exercise Physiology, Health Canada, and their agents assume no liability for persons who undertake physical activity, and if in doubt after completing this questionnaire, consult your doctor prior to physical activity.

No changes permitted. You are encouraged to photocopy the PAR-Q but only if you use the entire form.

Figure 3.6. Physical Activity Readiness Questionnaire (PAR-Q), p.1. (Source: Physical Activity Readiness Questionnaire (PAR-Q) © 2002. Used with permission from the Canadian Society for Exercise Physiology www.csep.ca.)

signs/symptoms related to the following: 1) blood profiles, medications; 2) anthropometrics (height and weight); or 3) blood pressure.

Budget Evaluation Plan Developing a budget prior to starting your health promotion program will allow you to plan ahead and ensure that you have the necessary resources. Your health promotion program budget may include such items as salaries, program materials, administrative needs, outside vendors, evaluations, and the costs associated with incentives used to drive participation.

Specifically, creating the budget for a health promotion project requires consideration of several items. These items consist of the following: personnel, consultant costs (e.g., training, evaluation), equipment (e.g., exercise balls, bands, blood pressure cuff, heart rate monitor), supplies (e.g., participants' notebook, paper), travel (e.g., training, conference), alterations, renovations, and contractual costs. Your broadest categories are related to expenditures and revenues. *Expenditures* include fixed or variable items as well as direct or indirect expenses. *Fixed expenditures* do not vary with the number of individuals served (e.g., rent, salaries for personnel, insurance costs). *Variable expenditures*, however, vary with the number of individuals served (e.g., copies of the handouts, program advertising, refreshments). *Direct costs* can include line items, such as staff, program coordinator, and materials or supplies. *Indirect costs* are not associated with the delivery of the program, but indirect costs are used in general to support the program. These items include costs associated with utilities, telephone, staff travel to attend training, clerical support staff, and office equipment. *Revenues* are funds that are obtained from grants and charitable fund raising. State or federal agencies sometimes match local dollars allocated to the health program. Last, you should include in-kind donations, such as, volunteer time, staff time, and printing, so that you can account for all of the expenses related to your program.

During the evaluation process, a comprehensive budget is essential because program costs are compared with outcomes. Ten to twenty percent of your budget should be alloted to the evaluation plan. See Figure 3.7 for a sample budget.

Developing a Sample Program Timeline

Now that we have reviewed all of the necessary pieces for developing your health promotion program, you may want to revisit your sample timeline (see Figure 2.3 and Figure 2.4). As you conduct your needs assessment; this is also the time to 1) convene program planning group, 2) review organizational policies for health promotion and share with stakeholders, and 3) conduct the Health Matters Assessment of Need (HMAN) and Health Matters Assessment of Capacity (HMAC) (see Appendix).

Beginning in Month 2, you can start thinking about developing your program. This is the time to start translating the assessment information into an action plan and objectives to share with stakeholders. You may also integrate *Health Matters: The Exercise and Nutrition Health Education Curriculum for People with Developmental Disabilities* (Marks, Sisirak, & Heller, 2010) into existing staff training and into new hire training (*optional*). A good time to advertise for program personnel is after 4 or 5 months. At Months 5 and 6, you can hire and train a program coordinator and advertise the health promotion program to stakeholders (people with

Organization name_____

| Detailed budget for initial budget period Direct costs only. | | | | From | | Through | |

PERSONNEL (Applicant organization only)		Type (Appointment) (months)	% Effort on the project	Instituti- onal base salary	Dollar amount requested (omit cents)		
Name	Role on project				Salary requested	Fringe benefits	Total
	Project coordinator						
SUBTOTALS				⟶			

Consultant costs
(e.g., training, evaluation)

Equipment (Itemize)
(e.g., exercise balls, bands, blood pressure cuff, heart rate monitor)

Supplies (Itemize by category)
(e.g., participants' notebooks, paper)

Travel
(e.g., training, conference, etc.)

Alterations and renovations (Itemize by category)

Other expenses (Itemize by category)

Consortium contractual costs	Direct costs	
Subtotal direct costs for initial budget period		$

Consortium/contractual costs	Facilities and administrative costs	
TOTAL DIRECT COSTS FOR INITIAL BUDGET PERIOD		$

Figure 3.7. Sample budget.

Adapted from National Institutes of Health. (2009). *Detailed budget for initial budget period.* Retrieved Jan. 2, 2010, from grants.nih.gov/grants/funding/phs398/fp4.doc. Copyright 2009 © by National Institutes of Health.

In *Health Matters for People with Developmental Disabilities: Creating a Sustainable Health Promotion Program,* by Beth Marks, Jasmina Sisirak, & Tamar Heller (2010, Paul H. Brookes Publishing Co.)

disabilities and staff). At Months 6 and 7, you can begin to train program personnel (staff). Baseline evaluation, including the health provider's consent, psychosocial survey, and fitness test for people with DD can be done at Months 7 and 8.

During Months 8 through 10, you can anticipate implementing the health promotion program. At the conclusion of the program, begin your post-project evaluations (e.g., psychosocial survey and fitness test for persons with DD). Also, collect staff and participant feedback about the program, and conduct process evaluation.

Last, you will want to analyze evaluation data at Month 11 and prepare a report in production during your final month. Once you have the report, you can disseminate the report both internally and externally. As you get feedback following your report, you can continue to discuss future directions and develop plans for sustaining your health promotion program.

Summary

This chapter identified strategies for setting realistic goals for your health promotion program. Organization goals and tools that support healthy lifestyles for adults with DD and their support people within organizations were provided. We also presented strategies for developing mutual goals. Last, we presented a sample budget and timeline for designing a program plan to implement a physical activity and health education program.

4

Implementing a Health Promotion Program

This chapter will help you design and implement a health promotion program tailored to your organizational needs that will encourage and support individuals with DD to become more physically active and make healthy food choices. In this chapter, we discuss the necessary components to implement a program plan for a physical activity and health education program for adults with DD.

Health Promotion Program Essentials

Health promotion programs should consist of creative outreach efforts, targeted health education activities, and assessment of preventive/screening interventions. You should think about incorporating and/or adapting existing health promotion curricula that have been developed and tested with people with disabilities to fit you health promotion program needs. For example, *Health Matters: The Exercise and Nutrition Health Education Curriculum for People with Developmental Disabilities* (Marks et al., 2010) and *Steps to Your Health*, part of the South Carolina Disabilities and Health Project (Mann, Zhou, McDermott, & Poston, 2006; Marks, Heller, Sisirak, Hsieh, & Pastorfield, 2005; Marks, Sisirak, Heller, & Riley, 2006), have been used with individuals with disabilities.

Implementation of health promotion programs in community settings beyond day/residential programs for people with DD is a critical step toward full community inclusion. Although community organizations are increasingly recognizing the benefits of health promotion and disease prevention for people living with long-term disabilities, developing and implementing accessible programs remains a challenge. Innovative community and worksite health promotion programs may include content related to obtaining health care services, making healthy food choices, and increasing physical activity

> *Although community organizations are increasingly recognizing the benefits of health promotion and disease prevention for adults living with long-term disabilities, developing and implementing accessible programs remains a challenge.*

and improving fitness levels. This requires developing methods of training staff in CBOs and recreation centers (e.g., YMCA, local park districts) and setting up on-site health promotion programs.

Health Promotion Program Components

Although few evidence-based, community programs aimed at achieving long-term lifestyle changes exist, preliminary studies (Heller, Marks, Pastorfield, Sisirak, & Hsieh, 2006; Marks et al., 2007; Marks, Sisirak, & Heller, 2008; Marks, Sisirak, & Hsieh, 2008) demonstrate the power of staff involvement and organizational support in the provision of health promotion activities to people with DD. Researchers at The University of Illinois at Chicago (UIC) have developed a Health Matters Train-the-Trainer Health Promotion Program for staff in community-based organizations to enhance health status, increase physical activity, and improve food choices in settings in which people work and live. Staff in the intervention group received an 8-hour, small-group (7–10 staff members), on-site Health Matters Train-the-Trainer Workshop. The training was given to staff immediately before they started the 12-week health promotion program for adults with DD. Technical assistance from UIC research team was provided to staff throughout the duration of the 12-week program via telephone, e-mail, and site visits. The goals of Health Matters Train-the-Trainer Program were the following: 1) Start and implement a physical activity and health education program using *Health Matters: The Exercise and Nutrition Health Education Curriculum for People with Developmental Disabilities* (Marks et al., 2010), 2) learn how to motivate and engage adults with DD in physical activity and health education, 3) teach core concepts related to physical activity and nutrition to adults with DD (e.g., heart rate, blood pressure, use of equipment, safety), and 4) support adults with DD to incorporate physical activities and healthy lifestyles into activities of daily living. The results from the Health Matters Program demonstrated the efficacy of a community-based health promotion program through significant changes in psychosocial health status, including less perceived pain, increased self-efficacy, and increased social/environmental health among participants with DD in the health promotion program compared with participants with DD in a comparison group who did not participate in the health promotion program (Marks et al., 2006). Staff who supported individuals participating in the Health Matters Program also showed significant changes in psychosocial health status, including an increase in vitality and energy, less fatigue, psychological well-being, less perceived pain, and increased exercise outcome expectations (Marks et al., 2007).

The goals that were incorporated in the Health Matters Program consisted of the following: 1) improve flexibility, aerobic capacity, balance, and strength; 2) increase knowledge about healthy lifestyles; and 3) teach staff and caregivers how to support participants to achieve these goals. The exercise classes included the following objectives:

- 1 hour of physical activity 3 days/week to improve fitness
- Emphasis on flexibility, cardiovascular endurance, balance, and muscle strength
- Safe use of the equipment and proper technique for exercises

The health education classes were integrated with the exercise classes. Health education classes include 37 interactive lessons in *Health Matters: The Exercise and Nutrition Health Education Curriculum for People with Developmental Disabilities* (Marks et al., 2010).

Designing an Accessible Exercise and Health Education Program

In working with people who have a variety of disabilities, several issues may require you to modify your teaching strategies. Areas of concern may include communication and speech (e.g., people may use augmentative communication devices), energy or stamina, hearing, learning or memory, mental health issues (mood, behavioral), mobility, and vision. As you teach the health education and exercise classes, you may consider the following questions:

1. *How will you set up the content incorporating principles of Universal Design (e.g., inclusive design) to ensure inclusion of all users including people with severe/profound intellectual disabilities and people with a variety of physical disabilities?* Universal Design aims to create communication, products, and environments to be maximally usable by all people, without adaptation or specialized design. The underlying premise is the following: If it works well for people across the spectrum of functional ability, it will work better for everyone. The usability of a communication strategy, product, or environment can be enhanced by including designs for a broad range of users that incorporate the five senses: seeing, touching, smelling, tasting, and hearing.

2. *What physical/environmental modifications will you need to make in the program to meet everyone's needs?*

3. *What communication strategies will you use to incorporate principles of Universal Design for people with DD and people with a range of intellectual and physical disabilities?*

Content modifications need to be made in the spirit of not disadvantaging, stigmatizing, or privileging any group of participants. Rather, teaching strategies are aimed at providing the same means of use for all participants. It's important to make the exercise and health education program appealing for all participants. For example, the following strategies can be used throughout the classes to accommodate a wide range of individual preferences and participants' functional abilities:

- Use pictures explaining both the exercise classes and the health education components.

- Limit the use of open-ended questions. Sometimes giving participants an option between two choices is a better way of getting responses from people. Giving people too many choices can be confusing. Provide yes or no questions with pictures. Or use either/or questions and provide two options in a question.

- Provide pictures of people doing health-promoting activities. Have the words cut out and available for participants to choose and describe.

- Include consistent reminders about previous classes.

- Limit the length of the session to 30 minutes.

- For participants who have limited range of motion, consider getting a physical therapy evaluation before starting to stretch participants on any regular basis. For some people with restricted range of motion, it may be helpful to have a physical therapist, parent, or doctor show how you move people through ranges of motion.

- Depending on the group, it may sometimes be useful to put people together with similar physical abilities. This is especially useful if participants are trying to learn how to do certain exercises or activities and other people who share their disability status can serve as role models. In addition, if the health education classes are discussing specific issues related to certain types of disabilities (e.g., Down syndrome, spina bifida, cerebral palsy), it can be helpful to have a group with similar types of disabilities or levels of functioning.

- Use content that is easy to understand regardless of participants' experience, knowledge, and language skills or concentration level.

- Develop more interactive goals for the program using pictures. For example, consider using pictures to delineate the goals for the Physical Activity Observation Sheet (PAOS; see Figure 4.1).

- Use more visual aids. Use pictures from magazines (e.g., photos of people with disabilities doing health-promoting activities).

- It may be useful to assume that most people are nonreaders or nonwriters, and ask participants if they would like assistance to fill out forms or complete health education activities.

- Consistently ask all participants if they would like assistance during the health education and fitness classes.

- Include more pictures of food items as you teach information on healthy eating. Also use real food products along with pictures. This is helpful for all participants.

- Create newsletters to summarize content. Include photos of participants and have them help develop the newsletter and make suggestions.

- Use familiar pictures from magazines, television, or the Internet as a way to reinforce educational messages related to health, nutrition, and physical activity.

- Incorporate sensory health messages (e.g., cut out pictures, draw grapes).

- Consider repeating one theme throughout the day in different programs, not just in the health promotion classes.

- Have staff be clear on their roles in promoting participants' health. Everyone has a role to play.

- In handouts, reduce the number of pictures on a page (e.g., consider having one picture per page plus real products, integrating artwork and skill building), for example, pick photos of grapes and show them to participants, have participants draw the grapes, show participants the real grapes, and then have participants eat the grapes.

- Use video clips to convey some of the many benefits physical activity can bring to a person with a DD. For example, the National Center on Physical Activity and Disability (NCPAD) presents an exercise video produced for individuals with DD as an example of how to use exercise bands for strength training among adults with DD (see http://www.ncpad.org).

PHYSICAL ACTIVITY OBSERVATION SHEET

Date_____   Session #_____

Interviewer_____   Weight_____

Ask the following questions (circle yes or no)

1)   Did you **sleep** last night?   Yes   No

2)   Have you been **sick** today?   Yes   No

3)   Did you **eat** breakfast and lunch?   Yes   No

4)   Did you take your **medication(s)**?   Yes   No

5)   Have your **medications changed**?   Yes   No
        (amount or type of medication)_____

        _____

6)   Do you have any **pain** today?   Yes   No
        Where is your pain?_____

        _____

7)   Overall, how are you **feeling** today?_____

8)   In general, how does he/she **look**? (e.g., pale, tired, sleepy, agitated)

        _____

        _____

	Pre–Exercise	Post–Exercise
Blood pressure (BP)		
Heart rate (HR)		
Blood sugar (only if participant has diabetes)		

(continued)

Figure 4.1.   Physical Activity Observation Sheet (PAOS).

Figure 4.1.   *(continued)*

Flexibility Training

Completed stretches for shoulders, arms, back/torso, hamstrings, quadriceps, calves?

(Circle response.)   Yes   No

Aerobic Training

(Circle response.)   Yes   No

Exercise modality	Exercise workload	HR: _____ minutes	HR: _____ minutes	HR: _____ minutes	Total time	Exercise BP

Target Heart Rate Range (THR): _____ bpm

Total exercise time: _____

Balance Training

Completed balance exercises? **(Circle response.)**   Yes   No

Strength Training

(Circle response.)   Yes   No

Modality	Recommended weight	Actual weight	Recommended repetitions	Actual repetitions

* When 20 repetitions are done comfortably (easily), increase weight by 10%

- For physical and environmental modification, you should aim for universal access. The first necessary step toward effective accommodations in your health education and fitness program is making sure that all obstacles, including stairs, narrow entryways, desks at the wrong height, and inaccessible washrooms are removed for people who use assistive devices or who have mobility concerns.

> It's important to make the exercise and health education program appealing for all participants.

Incorporating Flexibility, Aerobic, Balance, and Strength Exercises into Your Health Promotion Program

A thorough exercise program includes the following components of training: flexibility, aerobic, balance, and strength (FABS; see Appendix C of *Health Matters: The Exercise and Nutrition Health Education Curriculum for People with Developmental Disabilities*, Marks et al., 2010). Each component has a unique set of benefits and guidelines for maximum effectiveness. In developing your program, you may consider the Frequency, Intensity, Type, and Time (FITT) Principle as a guideline for planning. This principle outlines the necessary considerations for physical activities. Each letter represents a requirement for the activity to be safe and effective, as explained here:

F   Frequency: Number of times per week

I   Intensity: The difficulty level

T   Type: The type of exercise

T   Time: Length of each session

The following sections detail the use of the FITT Principle for each of the four main exercise components.

Flexibility Exercises

Flexibility refers to how far and how easily you can move your joints. As you get older, your tendons and other connective tissues around your muscles begin to shorten and tighten, restricting the movement of your joints—you become less flexible. In many cases this loss of mobility/flexibility is more related to inactivity than the aging process. The less you move, the less you're able to move. Being flexible has several health benefits, including helping prevent muscular aches and pains, improving posture and reducing neck and lower back discomfort, promoting greater flexibility, revitalizing the mind, reducing fatigue and increasing energy, and relieving stress and tension.

Although stretching is often a neglected component of an exercise program, it is important to include stretching at the beginning and at the end of each exercise session. At a minimum, everyone should stretch at the end of an exercise session.

When performing flexibility exercises, use the FITT Principle to the following specifications:

Frequency: Daily or just after exercise

Intensity: Only very mild discomfort in muscle that is being stretched

Type: Stretching and holding

Time: Hold each stretch for at least 15 seconds. You can also hold for more than 30 seconds.

Aerobic Exercises

In doing aerobic exercises, we keep our whole body moving fast enough to increase our heart rate and long enough so that our body has to use more oxygen. The goal of aerobic exercise is to strengthen our cardiovascular system (our heart, lungs, and blood vessels). Aerobic exercise is of benefit to us in that it can lower cholesterol, lower blood pressure and resting heart rate, control blood sugar, improve the immune system, and help to decrease excess body fat. Aerobic exercise can also revitalize the mind, reduce fatigue, and increase energy.

When performing aerobic exercises, use the FITT Principle to the following specifications:

Frequency: Between 3 to 5 days per week (in some cases, up to 6 days can be done)

Intensity: Based on either heart rate (to calculate target heart rate, see Figure 4.2) or perceived exertion (i.e., how difficult you think the physical activity is, see Figure 4.3)

Type: Using machines (e.g., treadmills, stair climbers), walking, jogging, cycling, or taking exercise classes. The cardiovascular component has three distinct segments. The first component is the warm-up. The purpose of warm-up is to prepare the body for exercise and should last for 5–10 minutes. It raises body temperature, heart rate, and breathing rate for the same reason that we allow

---

Male: 220 – age = Maximum heart rate   Female: 226 – age = Maximum heart rate

Calculating Target Heart Rate for exercise
Beginner: 50%–60% of maximum heart rate
Intermediate: 61%–70% of maximum heart rate
Advanced: 71%–80% of maximum heart rate

Calculating Target Heart Rate zone example:
Calculate beginner (50%–60%) target heart rate for Judy. Judy is a 26-year-old female.

226–26=200 (maximum heart rate)

Beginner Target Heart Rate
200 x 0.50 = 100
200 x 0.60 = 120

Answer: Judy's heart rate should be between 100–120 beats per minute during exercise.

Figure 4.2.   Target heart rate zone. (*Source:* American College of Sports Medicine, 2006).

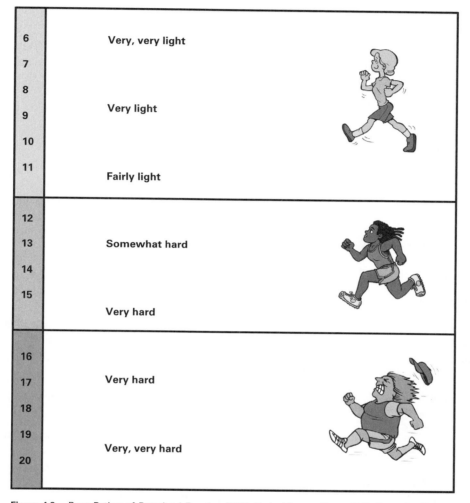

Borg Rating of Perceived Exertion Scale

Participants should be working at 12–13 (somewhat hard).

6	**Very, very light**
7	
8	**Very light**
9	
10	
11	**Fairly light**
12	
13	**Somewhat hard**
14	
15	**Very hard**
16	
17	**Very hard**
18	
19	**Very, very hard**
20	

Figure 4.3.   Borg Rating of Perceived Exertion (RPE) Scale (*Source:* Borg, 1998. From Marks, B., Sisirak, J., & Heller, T. [2010]. *Health matters: The exercise and nutrition health education curriculum for people with developmental disabilities* [p. 20]. Baltimore: Paul H. Brookes Publishing Co; reprinted by permission.).

our cars to warm up on a January morning in Chicago; our bodies (and our cars) function better when they are warmed up. The second component is the exercise component. The goal is to maintain our target heart rate for a minimum of 20 continuous minutes. Remember, if participants are not capable of completing 20 continuous minutes, break the session into short, multiple bouts. The cool-down follows the exercise component, and should last for 5–10 minutes. The cool-down helps the body transition from exercise to rest. During the cool-down, heart rate and blood pressure will decrease.

Time: For general fitness, work up to at least 20 minutes within target heart rate; can last for an hour or more. You can monitor intensity by using a heart rate monitor or by counting the pulse at wrist (radial pulse) or neck (carotid pulse). Do not press on both carotid arteries at the same time.

Balance Exercises

Balance exercises can help people with disabilities do the things that they like to do as they age. Exercises focused on improving balance can reduce the risk of falls. Balance exercises are nice in that you can develop a plan with participants that will allow them to do them almost anytime, anywhere, and as often as they like.

When performing balance exercises, use the FITT Principle to the following specifications:

Frequency: Daily or as a part of your exercise program

Intensity: Balance exercises can increase in difficulty, with exercises becoming more difficult as balance improves. For example, the same exercise becomes progressively harder with arms in any position, then with arms close to the body, and then with arms close to the body and holding a weight.

Type: Balance exercises that use sensory and motor systems

Time: For each balance exercise, repeat 8–15 times.

Strength Exercises

Strength and endurance exercises help our muscles to be able to move our bodies and other objects (e.g., pushing heavy furniture, carrying groceries up the stairs). Improving strength is beneficial in a variety of areas. For example, strength training can provide the following benefits:

- Increases metabolism. Strength training increases the body's metabolic rate, causing the body to burn more calories throughout the day.

- Increases bone density and prevents bone loss. Inactivity and aging can lead to a decrease in bone density and brittleness. Studies (Beck & Snow, 2003; Drinkwater, 1994; National Osteoporosis Foundation, n.d.; Wolff, van Croonenborg, Kemper, Kostense, & Twisk, 1999) have shown that consistent strength training can increase bone density and prevent osteoporosis.

- Increases lean muscle mass and muscle strength, power, and endurance

- Prevents injury by strengthening muscles

- Improves balance, flexibility, mobility, and stability (which means more comfortable living and fewer falls or accidents)

- Decreases the risk of heart disease

- Decreases cholesterol and lowers your blood pressure

- Revitalizes the mind, reduces fatigue, and increases energy

- Makes activities of daily living easier, such as rising from a chair

When performing strength exercises, use the FITT Principle to the following specifications:

Frequency: Two to three nonconsecutive days per week

Intensity: If you are using exercise machines and a pretest was completed (please see One-Repetition Maximum Test section), then begin training with 70% of pretest weight. Over the course of 1–2 week(s), increase resistance by 10%. Then ask the participant to lift the weight. If the participant can lift the weight for the desired number of repetitions with good form, increase the weight until the last repetition is somewhat difficult to lift. Order the exercises from using large muscle groups to small muscle groups: Progress by increasing repetitions (number of times the weight is lifted) before adding resistance (weight). Once the participant can complete 15 repetitions with good form, increase resistance. The amount depends on the participant and the exercise. The last repetition should be somewhat hard to complete.

Type: Machines, free weights, elastic bands, milk jugs full of water

Time: For general fitness, exercise is recommended to last 30–60 minutes, or one set of 8 to 12 repetitions. A *repetition* is lifting and lowering the weight once and a *set* is a predetermined number of repetitions.

Helpful Tips for your Health Promotion Program

Health promotion programs should be safe, fun, progressive in nature, and designed with the participant's goals in mind. Here are some helpful tips to keep in mind when preparing your health promotion program.

For the first 2 weeks of the program, participants will start with 30–40 minutes per session and will increase to 1-hour sessions at the beginning of the third week. During the first 2 weeks of the exercise program, participants will become familiar with the equipment and will determine what exercises they want to perform. If a participant misses a session, he or she will have the opportunity for make-up sessions the following week by going an extra day. When make-ups occur, the exercise will be less intense because the participant will be exercising for 2 consecutive days.

> A moderate *level of activity is needed to achieve health benefits. Participants can elect to do more if they are physically capable of doing so.*

The intensity level of the physical activity should be geared to the participant's initial fitness level. Every attempt should be made to adhere to the guidelines established by the American College of Sports Medicine and the Surgeon General's Report on Physical Activity and Health (American College of Sports Medicine, 2006), which states that a *moderate* level of activity is needed to achieve health benefits. Participants can elect to do more if they are physically capable of doing so.

The exercises should vary according to participants' preferences. For example, in the aerobic area, activities may include walking, stationary cycling, Nu-step recumbent stepping (sitting and moving arms and legs together), stepping exercises, arm ergometry, and low-impact aerobics. In the area of strength, participants can perform calisthenics such as wall push-ups and modified sit-ups, and participants can also use a variety of smaller pieces of equipment, such as elastic tubing.

The following list contains more helpful tips to keep in mind:

1. If a cardiovascular exercise test is performed, use maximum heart rate attained for the target heart rate calculation.

2. Use percent of heart rate or target heart rate (THR, see Figure 4.2) method to determine exercise level. Always use the low end of the recommended range for people who are sedentary.

3. Begin cardiovascular session with a 5-minute warm-up.

4. After the warm-up, begin to increase the intensity to get heart rate within the desired range (e.g., for biking exercises, increase resistance or speed of pedaling; for treadmill, increase the speed or elevation; for a stepper, increase the rate of stepping or height of step).

5. Monitor heart rate as often as possible. If heart rate increases over recommended range, decrease intensity, lower grade, or lower speed.

6. Use an interval program (e.g., circuit training, where participants are doing different types of exercises for a shorter amount of time) for those with low levels of fitness.

7. Always end the program with a cool-down of at least 5 minutes. For participants on ACE inhibitors (**A**ngiotensin-**C**onverting **E**nzymes are a group of medications used primarily in treatment of *hypertension* and *congestive heart failure*) or nitrates, the cool-down must be extended to 10 minutes.

8. Progress by increasing length or intensity of the session. Once a participant can complete 30 minutes at the low end of his or her target heart rate, then increase target heart rate by five beats per minute.

Sample Agenda for the Exercise Portion of Your Health Promotion Program

- Begin with a group warm-up session.

- Continue with a group stretching session.

- Divide group between strength and cardiovascular training areas.

- Alternate or switch groups (e.g., strength goes to cardiovascular and cardiovascular goes to strength).

- Complete a group cool-down session.

- Conclude with a group stretching session. By spending 10 to 15 minutes to slow down body movements, muscles can cool off and problems related to dizziness can be avoided. This is also a time to give muscles a chance to get rid of lactic acid build-up. It's important to avoid stopping suddenly or worse, sitting down, right after a workout!

Recommended Supplies for
Your Health Promotion Program

We recommend several items that can be used to monitor health-related changes among participants. The purpose of monitoring health is twofold. First, monitoring health provides immediate feedback for support people to see how participants are doing. For example, some participants may seem as though they are not exercising very strenuously, when in fact their heart rates may be quite elevated as they are starting at a low level of conditioning. Conversely, participants may also be expressing significant distress as they start to sweat. But their heart rates may have only increased from 72 beats per minute to 76 beats per minute. Knowing participants' heart rates gives staff assurance that each participant is exercising within a safe zone.

> *Allowing participants to monitor their heart rate and blood pressure will allow them to see how they can change their blood pressure and heart rate through physical activity and healthy food choices.*

Second, heart rate and blood pressure monitoring provides tangible feedback for participants as to how they are doing. We have found this to be quite motivating for participants. The intent is not to "medicalize" the exercise program, rather the intent is to give participants greater control in beginning to understand the relationship between their exercise and their blood pressure and heart rate. Allowing participants to monitor their heart rate and blood pressure will allow them to see how they can change their blood pressure and heart rate through physical activity and healthy food choices.

We recommend several items that can be used to monitor health-related changes among participants, such as a heart rate monitor, a blood pressure monitor, a blood sugar monitor (if a participant has diabetes), and a personal notebook. We also recommend that participants complete a PAOS (see Figure 4.1) before beginning their health promotion program.

Heart Rate Monitor

Although using a heart rate monitor is not necessary for everyone, it is a great tool for exercisers. Even if used temporarily, it will help a participant learn how he or she feels at a given heart rate and may allow that participant to become a better judge of his or her exercise tolerance and any limitations. Heart rate monitors are also useful for new exercisers because the devices help these individuals set limits and monitor their progress. It is important for participants to pay attention to their bodies and not rely solely on the monitor for feedback; however, a heart rate monitor is never a bad idea. Many people like a heart rate monitor because it helps them stay interested in their exercise, and it helps them monitor their progress on a daily basis. We have found that the Polar Heart Rate Monitors (http://www.polarusa.com) are durable and effective. In particular, we have found that the basic, one-button watch is the easiest heart rate monitor to use.

Understanding Heart Rate for Use with the Heart Rate Monitor

Normal heart rate is 60–90 beats per minute. Heart rate can be affected by a variety of factors, including the following:

- Cardiovascular fitness, age, and hormones can affect your HR.

- Use of medications may speed up or slow down your HR.

- Caffeine and cigarettes speed up your HR.

- Stress can increase your HR.

- Body temperature can affect your HR (hot—HR elevated, cold—HR lowered).

- Dehydration can increase HR.

- Different illnesses, health conditions, general health status and emotional state can affect your HR.

During exercise, it is important to monitor heart rate because heart rate typically increases during any physical activity or exercise. Moreover, how hard a person exercises is reflected in his or her heart rate. The harder a person exercises, the higher the heart rate. Because hard work alone does not guarantee better results, it is important to exercise within a personal THR (see Figure 4.2 for information on how to calculate a THR). In working with participants with disabilities, we have found that most people will begin an exercise program at a beginner level. Use Figure 4.2 to see how to calculate target heart rate zones for exercising.

Blood Pressure Monitor

Blood pressure typically increases during physical activity. However, in the long term, any exercise will help lower your blood pressure. When choosing the blood pressure monitor, we have found that wrist monitors are good to use with participants. Unlike the upper arm, electronic blood pressure cuffs, the wrist monitors can be used with participants who range in weight, wrist, and arm size. They are also easy for participants to use.

Understanding Blood Pressure for Use with the Blood Pressure Monitor

Blood pressure is blood flow through your heart. Blood pressure is measured by reading two numbers. One number refers to the beating of the heart (systolic), and the other number refers to the heart relaxing (diastolic). That is, systolic blood pressure (SBP) is the maximum pressure exerted when the heart contracts, and diastolic blood pressure (DBP) is the pressure in the arteries (walled vessels that carry blood from the heart through the body) when the heart is at rest.

A normal blood pressure is below 120/80 millimeters of mercury (mm Hg), which is an SBP of 120 and DBP of 80. Making sure that our blood pressure is within normal limits is very important because maintaining a blood pressure in a healthy range can help prevent heart disease, kidney failure, eye complications, and other health problems. Untreated high blood pressure (or hypertension) can result in stroke.

Blood pressure is affected by the following:

- Medications can increase or decrease your BP.

- Physical activity and exercise can have positive or negative effects on BP.

Table 4.1. Blood pressure values for exercising

DBP	SBP		
	<120	120–139	>140
<80	Optimal	Prehypertension	High
80–89	Prehypertension	Prehypertension	High
>90	High	High	High

Normal values: 120/80 mm Hg (SBP/DBP)
DO NOT EXERCISE IF:
SBP is >200 mm Hg **or** DBP is >100 mm Hg
American Heart Association (n.d.). Blood pressure. Available at http://www.americanheart.org/presenter.jhtml?identifier=4473.

- Caffeine and cigarettes speed up your BP.

- Stress/anxiety increase your BP.

- Sleep can have positive and negative effects on BP.

- Relaxation can have a positive effect on BP.

- Different illnesses and health conditions affect BP.

- Diet can have positive or negative effects on BP.

- Atmospheric pressure can affect BP.

- Hardening of the arteries increases BP.

- Standing up too fast can make your BP drop.

Any exercise will help lower your blood pressure. Endurance exercises, such as walking, jogging, swimming, stair climbing, and bike riding can help control blood pressure. Even weight lifting can be used to treat high blood pressure. Practically any exercise you can think of can be used to lower your blood pressure. Refer to Table 4.1 to see blood pressure values that are considered optimal, prehypertension, and high. A participant should not exercise if his or her SBP is >200 mm Hg *or* DBP is >100 mm Hg.

Blood Sugar Monitoring

Before a participant begins an exercise program, he or she must have approval from his or her health care provider. This includes knowing whether the individual has diabetes and will need to check his or her blood sugar prior to exercising. Table 4.2, Blood Sugar and Exercise, details a protocol that can be used if a participant has diabetes.

Personal Notebook for Participants

Each participant is encouraged to have his or her own personal notebook as he or she begins a health promotion program. Having a personal notebook can increase

Table 4.2. Blood sugar and exercise

- Before starting any new physical activity program, get your health care provider's OK to exercise.
- Exercise can help you improve your blood sugar control.
- Remember to check your blood sugar BEFORE, DURING, and AFTER exercise. This will help you track how your body responds to exercise and help you prevent rapid blood sugar changes.

Check your blood sugar BEFORE physical activity

Think about these general guidelines:

- **Lower than 100 milligrams per deciliter (mg/dL).** Your blood sugar is too low to exercise. Eat a small snack containing carbohydrates such as fruit or crackers before starting your exercise.
- **100 to 250 mg/dL.** For most people this is a safe blood sugar range. You may start your exercise!
- **250 mg/dL or higher.** Caution zone! Test your urine for ketones (compound made when your body breaks down fat for energy). Too many ketones indicate that your body doesn't have enough insulin to control blood sugar. Exercising with high level of ketones may lead to a serious health complication ketoacidosis that needs immediate treatment. Wait for the levels of ketones to come down before exercise.
- **300 mg/dL or higher.** Do not exercise! Your blood sugar may be too high and is putting you at risk for ketoacidosis. Wait for the levels of ketones to come down before exercise.

Watch for symptoms of low blood sugar DURING physical activity

Your blood sugar may change during exercise. If you are feeling shaky, dizzy, faint, confused, or have changes in coordination or vision, stop exercising and eat or drink something to raise your blood sugar level. Check your blood sugar and recheck it again 15 minutes later after your snack.

Check your blood sugar AFTER physical activity

After exercise, check your blood sugar immediately. Exercise uses up reserve sugar stored in your liver and muscles. Your body will rebuild these stores by taking sugar from your blood. The longer you exercise, the longer your blood sugar will be affected.

Sources: Mayo Clinic (n.d.). *Diabetes and exercise: When to monitor your blood sugar.* Available at http://www.mayoclinic.com/health/diabetes-and-exercise/DA00105; National Institute of Diabetes and Digestive and Kidney Diseases. http://diabetes.niddk.nih.gov/dm/pubs/physical_ez/index.htm

participants' involvement and feelings of ownership in the program. Personalizing each notebook by inserting a digital photo of each participant encourages ownership and engagement in the exercise and health education program. The personal notebook can include a goals worksheet that can be used to develop goals with each participant during the first class session of the program. Refer back to Chapter 3, Figure 3.3, for My Goals for the Program Form for a sample goals worksheet. The goals of the program may be reviewed occasionally during the program so that participants can be reminded of their goals. It is important to note that individual goals may be revised and changed during the program. This sheet can also be used for staff to develop their own goals for the program.

After you have developed your program, we recommend including the PAOS in your participants' personal notebook (see Figure 4.1) to determine a participant's readiness for physical activity before each session. PAOS can also be used as a teaching and motivational tool for participants. The PAOS form can be used before every exercise class. Using PAOS with participants is a useful way to engage participants in a discussion about key concepts related to exercise and physical activity.

The Borg Rating of Perceived Exertion (RPE) Scale (see Figure 4.3) should also be included in the personal notebook. Perceived exertion is how hard you feel your body is working. It is based on the physical sensations a person experiences during physical activity, including increased heart rate, increased breathing rate, increased sweating, and muscle fatigue. Although this is a subjective measure, a person's exertion rating may provide a fairly good estimate of the actual heart rate during physical activity. Perceived exertion ratings between 12 and 14 on the Borg RPE Scale suggest that physical activity is being performed at a moderate level of intensity. The Borg RPE Scale should be used with people that are using medications that decrease their heart rate, such as beta blockers.

The Borg RPE Scale is also a useful tool to be used along with a heart rate monitor to gauge heart rate and show a participant how hard he or she is exercising. For example, if a participant is saying that he or she is working very hard (16–20 rating), and his or her heart rate has not even reached his or her target heart rate zone, you may show the participant what his or her actual heart rate is and how far he or she has to go to reach the target zone. Remember, medication can affect exercise. Some people who take beta blocker medication and exercise describe the sensation of exercising as "walking through the mud." A person may feel slowed down due to the beta blockers even though he or she is working hard. This is because medication is trying to decrease heart rate while exercise is trying to increase it.

Through the experience of monitoring how a person's body feels it will become easier to know when to adjust the intensity of exercise. For example, a participant who wants to engage in moderate-intensity activity would aim for a Borg RPE level of "somewhat hard," or 12–14 on the Borg RPE Scale. If the participant describes his or her muscle fatigue and breathing as "very light," or 9 on the Borg RPE Scale, he or she would want to increase exercise intensity. Futhermore, if the participant felt his or her exertion was "extremely hard," or 19 on the Borg RPE Scale, he or she would need to slow down his or her movements to achieve moderate-intensity range.

Checklist for Getting Started

The following is a sample checklist that will help you get started with your health promotion program. This checklist was adapted using a list developed by ARCA, a community-based organization in New Mexico, as a tool to ensure readiness in starting a health promotion program. ARCA participated in the UIC's Health Matters program.

1. Make sure you have developed your program plan.

2. Obtain health care provider approval before starting any physical activity. Your caseworker can help.

3. Request baseline blood sugar and blood cholesterol measurements when asking for the health care provider's approval.

4. Coordinate FABS assessments at the beginning and the end of the program with coordinator.

5. Review the teaching lessons you will use (see *Health Matters: The Exercise and Nutrition Health Education Curriculum for People with Developmental Disabilities* [Marks et al., 2010] for a detailed curriculum of lessons to include in your health promotion program), and plan the first lesson. The curriculum is a 12-week, evidence-based health education program that incorporates approximately 1 hour of learning and 1 hour of exercise. We recommend having three

sessions weekly and that you assist your participants to record a PAOS in their personal notebooks for each class. There are 36 PAOS handouts, one per class.

6.   Gather materials and supplies (e.g., pens, copies of handouts, blackboard and chalk, heart rate and blood pressure monitors, Thera bands or weight bars).

7.   Start the first lesson/exercise session.

   a.   Have participants come prepared with a water bottle and appropriate footwear and clothing.

   b.   We recommend that participants not bring food or outside drink during class.

   c.   Have participants complete their PAOS and record blood pressure and heart rate.

   d.   Before the exercise component of the health promotion program, have participants put on their heart rate monitors or any other needed monitors to check their heart and/or blood pressure (*Tip:* Participants can slip heart rate monitors over their feet or head to avoid spending a lot of time fastening). Have participants with DD check and record blood pressure and heart rate. Keep track that your students are recording this information at each class—provide staff support as needed.

   e.   Begin educational lesson. Use open-ended questions to assess knowledge. Close educational component and begin exercise session.

   f.   Complete warm-ups and stretching activities first, then complete vigorous activity verified by the heart rate monitors and, finally, complete cool-down and stretching exercises.

   g.   Begin exercise component of the health promotion program. (*Tip:* When exercising, it is good to alternate strength training days with aerobic days.) Each participant should have a water bottle and appropriate footwear and clothing.

   h.   Have students check and record blood pressure and heart rate.

   i.   Break down, give reminders for next class.

   j.   Review today's key concepts at the start of the next class.

CASE SCENARIO

Creating a Space for Physical Activity

A community-based organization providing services to people with DD is planning to develop a new health promotion program. They have very limited resources—a room the size of an average classroom and no exercise equipment—but their staff is very interested in starting a program. The organization needs help to figure out how to develop a program with these limited resources.

Q1:   What plan should staff develop to address this issue?

Q2:   What barriers might be expected in implementing this plan?

Q3:   What are some potential resources that the management team can use to ensure the success of the proposed plan?

Sample Program

Exercise and Health Education Overview

The goal of a 12-week exercise and health education program is to support participants to identify exercises that they like to do and encourage them to gain a) knowledge, b) skills, and c) confidence in being able to exercise three days a week at a level of intensity tailored to their individual needs. *Health Matters: The Exercise and Nutrition Health Education Curriculum for People with Developmental Disabilities* (Marks et al., 2010) can be used to introduce core concepts related to physical activity, exercise, and nutrition (e.g., physical activity, energy, heart rate, blood pressure, hydration, medications, safety, breathing, good pain and bad pain, sleep and exercise) to participants with developmental disabilities, along with strategies for maintaining behavior and lifestyle changes. Along with the health education classes, 12-week exercise program can consist of the following activities: 1) Warm-ups; 2) FABS; and 3) Cool-Downs.

Warm-Ups: 5 minutes (e.g., jumping jacks, arm circles, seated leg circles)

FABS

> **Flexibility**—5 minutes (e.g., head tilts, shoulder stretch, trunk side bends, leg stretch, calf stretch)
> **Aerobic**—30 minutes (e.g., treadmill, bike, speed walk around gym)
> **Balance**—5 minutes (e.g., heal-to-toe walking, stand on one foot)
> **Strength**—20 minutes (e.g., wrist curls, bicep curls, arm raises, sit-to-stand, wall sits, plantar flexion)

Cool Downs: 5 minutes (e.g., walk around gym)

Safety and Physical Activity

Safety and physical activity can be a particular issue if you choose to use a lot of equipment (e.g., free weights, treadmills, other fitness center equipment). If choosing to do physical training in this environment, be sure to plan to have enough staff to assist and "spot" participants during the entire exercise session. For each exercise, demonstrate proper technique. If necessary, break the exercise into basic components.

Exercise Prescription Using the One-Repetition Maximum Test

If you are using weight machines, an exercise prescription can be calculated with the One-Repetition Maximum (1-RM) test. The 1-RM test is used to assess dynamic muscle strength. It measures the maximum amount of weight that can be lifted with good form. To complete this test, you will need to have access to the selected piece of gym equipment. You will also need an appropriate data sheet and pen. (See Figure 2.8 in Chapter 2.)

To prepare participants, you will need to explain to each participant what the test is and the purpose of that test, discuss any limitations or restrictions the participant may have in performing any of the tests, and always provide a demonstration for each participant. Ask the participant if he or she has any questions before he or she performs the 1-RM test.

To complete the 1-RM test, you should be familiar with the equipment and the correct form positioning before any testing; prepare the piece of equipment that the participant will be using; record position of seat, arm distance, or any placement that is unique to the participant (this will ensure that the participant gets tested with a proper form each time); and have at least one spotter for the participant. Have other spotters ready if a heavy 1-RM is anticipated.

The following instructions can be used with participants to do the 1-RM test:

1. Warm up with 5 to 10 repetitions at an easy weight (or 40%–60% of what you think the participant can lift). The participant will get used to the machine and learn the right form.

2. Rest for 1 minute while stretching.

3. Perform three to five repetitions at 60%–80% of the perceived maximum.

4. Increase the weight slightly. The participant should be at or close to the perceived 1-RM.

5. Increase the weight by increments (5–10 pounds) until the participant feels that they have reached the 1-RM. If the participant's arms or legs start shaking, and he or she is slowly lifting the weight, you have probably reached the maximum. Remember, the weight must be lifted with good form.

6. Record the 1-RM on the appropriate data sheet(s).

Plan for future lifting to involve an initial weight of 70% of the 1-RM test. When the participant can lift 20 repetitions comfortably (usually after 2 weeks), increase weight by 10%—this incremental increase is often referred to as the rule of 10%.

Summary

This chapter has helped you design a health promotion program designed with your organizational needs in mind. We discussed the necessary components to implement a program plan for a physical activity and health education program for adults with DD and provided a sample checklist for getting started. We also discussed safety and the use of monitoring systems.

Sustaining Your Health Promotion Program

This final chapter discusses strategies for keeping your health promotion program going. We discuss the role of culturally representative health promotion programming. In addition, we present health and wellness resources and provide motivational strategies that can be used over time to keep your program current and sustainable.

Culturally Representative Health Promotion Programming

Health promotion programs are dynamic endeavors. They change depending on the political and economical conditions, state and local environment, organizational and cultural shifts in leadership and staffing, and changes within the population that your organization supports. Once the process of developing a health promotion program is set in place and regular classes are held to teach people with DD how to increase physical activity, engage in fitness activities, and make healthy food choices, you may want to focus on evaluating your health promotion program outcomes. As seen earlier in Figure 2.6, the amount of effort decreases during this phase; however, this is a critical component for long-term success and sustainability. During this stage, you will want to examine various evaluation components of your organizational and health promotion program plan as were noted in Figures 2.5 and 2.7. For example, you may want to develop mechanisms for reporting your successes in terms of numbers of people (staff and clients) that were taught, number of classes held, and client outcome measures. Evaluation is a cyclical process that ensures that your program continues to be culturally responsive to the needs of your clients, employees, and organizational mission over time. This, in turn, results in sustainability.

Throughout this stage, soliciting staff and participant-with-DD feedback related to the health promotion program, understanding the processes of running a program (positive and negative), and sharing the outcomes and lessons learned with others internally and outside of your organization is important (see Figure 2.5).

Person-centered planning (PCP), introduced more than 20 years ago, was an innovative approach aimed at including individuals with DD by understanding their experiences and working with them and their supports (e.g., paid caregivers, family members, health care providers) to increase their quality of life (O'Brien, O'Brien, & Mount, 1997). Ways of listening and understanding an individual's health-related goals and the development of action plans and evaluation strategies can be included in this approach. PCP places social supports of caregivers, family, and friends at the center of these plans (Heller, Miller, et al., 2000; O'Brien et al., 1997).

By incorporating PCP principles within your health promotion program evaluation, you are fostering full participation among individuals with disabilities to maximize the spirit of self-determination. As we begin to focus on making health care and health promotion activities universally accessible for persons with disabilities, we can also support people to take a more active role in evaluating whether their health promotion services are *equitable, accessible, acceptable, available,* and *culturally relevant.* Encouraging participants with DD and employees to assume an active role in evaluating their health promotion program is a key component in motivating clients and employees. It is easy to motivate people when they see their successes in how they feel and look. As people feel better and have more energy, they are able to more actively participate in activities. Most people want to maintain healthy lifestyles, but the challenging part is maintaining the infrastructure of support.

> *Evaluation is a cyclical process that ensures that your program continues to be culturally responsive to the needs of your clients, employees, and organizational mission over time.*

Program Viability

We have found that one of the strengths in having a health promotion program for people with DD is its focused attention on giving participants the opportunity to be successful in being able to exercise and make healthy food choices. These successes often translate into individuals seeing and feeling changes in their bodies and in how they feel. As people move beyond action, supporting participants with DD to continue making long-term goals that incorporate restructuring the environment, getting back on track, and reviewing goals to stay connected is critical.

If you are using *Health Matters: The Exercise and Nutrition Health Education Curriculum for People with Developmental Disabilities* (Marks et al., 2010) as a part of your health promotion program, one way to keep your program viable and active is to incorporate the lessons in the Appendix titled "Lifelong Learning Series." These lessons were designed to complement the 37 lessons that were taught in *Health Matters.* The lessons were generated by people with DD and were created as a way of initiating and encouraging lifelong learning related to health and adoption of healthy lifestyles. Lessons include the themes of advocacy and social support, physical activity, nutrition, and general health. Specifically, the aim of the lessons is to reinforce the information presented during the program and to provide ongoing support for people to continue developing new skills and greater confidence to engage in regular physical activity and make healthy food choices. In addition, similar to the teaching strategies used in the core lessons, the concepts of choice, self-determination, self-efficacy, self-advocacy, and rights and responsibilities should be used as a foundation for all of the classes.

Strategies for Motivating Participants

Several strategies can be used to improve participation, including reminders and rewards and caregiver support. The following sections also include sample motivational strategies and important motivational tips.

Caregiver Support

Staff and family members can provide support for people with DD to engage in physical activity in a variety of ways. Role modeling is a critical key to changing any health behavior or maintaining healthy behaviors. Expecting people with DD to be physically active and make healthy food choices will be easier if they are surrounded by people who are physically active and who are eating nutritious foods. Support people can use a range of strategies to increase the participation of people with DD. For example, a support person can do the following activities:

1. Offer to exercise with the individual with DD.

2. Give him or her helpful reminders to exercise (e.g., "Are you going to exercise tonight?").

3. Give the individual encouragement to stick with his or her exercise program.

4. Discuss different types of exercise.

5. Discuss possible rewards for exercising.

6. Plan for physical activity on recreational outings.

7. Discuss ideas on ways to become more physically active.

8. Talk about what people like about exercising.

9. Take individuals with DD to another exercise program (*Note:* You may have to provide transportation).

10. Identify ways of paying for an exercise program.

11. Show individuals with DD how to exercise.

Furthermore, staff and family members can influence the nutrition choices of people with DD; they may be positive or negative role models or gatekeepers. Staff turnover may be a barrier to improved nutrition due to lack of training, education, and experience of new staff members. Dietary quality can also be directly influenced by the behavior of staff. For example, staff and family members can influence participants' choices in planning and preparing meals. Staff and family members can also facilitate access to snacks and foods and influence food choices. Staff and family members can also provide support in a variety of ways:

1. Encourage the individual with DD to avoid eating "unhealthy foods" (e.g., cake, chips).

2. Assist in developing plans and goals for changing eating habits.

3. Remind people not to eat high-fat, high-salt foods and to eat more fruits and vegetables.

4. Compliment an individual on changing his or her eating habits (e.g., "Keep it up," "We are proud of you").

5. Offer fruits and vegetables as a snack during the day.

Sample Motivational Strategies

One of the formidable challenges with any health promotion program is developing strategies aimed at keeping your program fresh and creative while maintaining safety. Furthermore, a health promotion program must be fun, must be progressive in nature (i.e., building on health knowledge that has already been learned or increasing the level of physical activity), and must include participants' goals. Maintaining safety requires consideration of the following for your participants with DD: 1) obtaining health provider approval to exercise, 2) knowing participant health conditions, and 3) understanding the medications that your participants are taking. The sample motivational strategies included in the next section can be used to develop innovative strategies for your program. These strategies have been used in community-based organizations as a way to keep health promotion programs viable and fun for participants (Mauer, personal communication, May 8, 2005). The goal of motivational strategies is to keep people interested, engaged, and feeling good about participating in the program.

What doesn't work:

- Negative attitudes

- Forcing people to work out

- Rushing people

- Disengaging yourself from the workout

What does work (activities for motivation):

- *Fitness raffle:* Selected individual with DD chooses exercises, sets, and repetitions.

- *Phone book game:* Class leader randomly flips through the phone book and selects a number (e.g., telephone number 305-7654 = 3 sets of 7 reps).

- *Bonus points frenzy game:* Offer points for things like highest calorie burner or being on time for class. Rewards can include being a fitness director or leading the group for a day. The individual gets to choose his or her favorite exercise or activity or selects the radio station for the workout session, or the individual gets to choose the most "coveted" exercise equipment or activity.

- *Flip the Script game:* "You're the boss for the day." Have a participant make the rules for things that can be "turned over" (e.g., change the order of the exercises).

- *Exercise contest:* Encourage a friendly exercise contest between individuals. (*Note:* The success of this game depends on the individuals involved.)

- *Location Change:* Change the location of the class if possible.

- *Fitness Passport–Exercise Around the World game:* Have a map of the world and give people a book for stamps. Participants can earn stamps when coming to the classes. With every three to six stamps (1–2 weeks of workout three times per week), individuals travel to a new country. With every country, people get a fitness-related gift (e.g., water bottle, T-shirt, fitness CD).

- *Free Day:* Give participants complete choice over activities.

Important Safety Tips

The following list of safety tips was developed by a community-based organization based on their experiences in developing a structured health promotion program within their organization (ARCA, 2005).

- Safety of those involved is always the first consideration.

- Form is critical to productive exercise.

- Monitor movements and have enough staff available to help with form as needed.

- Do *not* ask people to lift weights that are too heavy or off balance or to complete exercises if they cause pain.

- Exercise coordinators can provide many simple exercise routines for people who need to start more slowly.

- Music can help create rhythm during exercise.

- Remember—repetition helps, as does visual, verbal, and tactile prompts—so participants remember what you taught during the educational session.

- You may write down individual target heart rate zones on the back of participants' ID badge holders or make a clip with target heart rate zones that participants can wear while exercising. Participants may clip their ID badge holders to their workout clothes to be reminded of their personal target heart rate zone.

- There are many low-cost walking tapes that can be used in a pinch as an exercise session.

- If a staff scheduling problem arises, it's important to call the coordinator and try to have a substitute lead the class versus canceling the class altogether.

Remember: Keep it light, and allow for errorless learning. If you want folks to keep doing this, it has to be fun!

Getting Resources for Your Health Promotion Program

Identifying local community organizations for support of your health promotion program is one way of increasing the visibility and viability of your program for people with DD. Your local YMCA or park district is a good place to start developing a collaborative partnership. As a community-based organization that provides services to people with DD, you can work with your local recreation centers to improve and offer disability-friendly recreational services for people with DD. You can do cross-collaborative trainings with your local community recreational organizations and local community health services. These partnerships ensure that people with DD are actively engaged in developing cross-collaborative programs and are participating in mainstream community health and recreational activities. In addition, inviting other community members, such as health professionals, volunteers, and university students to serve as guest speakers during the health education sessions is another way of keeping the program innovative and progressive.

> *You can do cross-collaborative trainings with your local community recreational organizations and local community health services.*

The Rehabilitation Research and Training Center on Aging with Developmental Disabilities (RRTCADD; see http://www.rrtcadd.org) provides technical assistance on a range of topics, including Health Matters Train-the-Trainer Workshops, caregiver issues, and age-friendly environments. The RRTCADD promotes the successful aging of adults with intellectual and developmental disabilities in response to physical, cognitive, and environmental changes. Its coordinated research, training, and dissemination activities promote progressive policies and supports to maintain health and function, self-determination, independence, and active engagement in life. The RRTCADD is a national resource for researchers, people with intellectual and developmental disabilities, their families, service providers, policy makers, advocacy groups, students, and the general community.

Future Directions

As you document your successes with your participants who have disabilities, it is good to consider your next steps. Branding your health and wellness program is another strategy that can be helpful for seeking future funding and recognition within your local community. For example, giving a name and creating a logo for your new health promotion program may increase its visibility within the organization and your community. Make sure that you use the name and the logo when advertising, e-mailing, and posting flyers about health promotion activities. As you continue to evaluate and demonstrate your results, you want to secure a stable funding source for a coordinator of your health promotion program.

Another strategy to consider relates to employee health programs. As previously noted, many health promotion initiatives in the private sector have offered employees opportunities to engage in health promotion programs. For your organization, you may want to consider including or adding a health and wellness program for employees. The benefits of employee-based health programs can include the following:

1. A healthier workforce

2. Employees who can better serve as role models for clients with disabilities

3. Lower staff turnover

4. Reduced workers' compensation claims

5. Decrease in workers' compensation premiums

Ultimately, a healthy workforce will provide superior support services for people with DD, especially when supporting their participation in a health promotion program. These efforts and broad changes can in turn greatly enhance the health and well-being of individuals with DD for years to come.

Summary

This final chapter has helped you identify strategies for keeping your health promotion program for individuals with DD going. We discussed the role of culturally representative health promotion programming. To support your efforts, we presented community resources and provide motivational and safety strategies. We hope this book has provided you with the tools and resources to implement a sustainable health promotion program.

References

Ad Hoc Committee on Health Literacy for the Council on Scientific Affairs: American Medical Association. (1999). Health literacy: Report of the Council on Scientific Affairs. *JAMA: The Journal of the American Medical Association, 281*(6), 552–557.

Ailey, S.H., Miller, A.M., Heller, T., & Smith, E.V. (2006). Evaluating an interpersonal model of depression among adults with Down syndrome. *Research & Theory for Nursing Practice, 20*(3), 229–246.

Aldana, S.G. (1998). Financial impact of worksite health promotion and methodological quality of the evidence. *Art of Health Promotion, 2*(1), 1–8.

American Association on Mental Retardation. (2002). *Mental retardation: Definition, classification, and systems of support* (10th ed.). Washington, DC: Author.

American College of Sports Medicine. (2006). *ACSM's guidelines for exercise testing and prescriptions* (7th ed.). Indianapolis: Author.

American Heart Association. (2010). *Women, heart disease and stroke*. Retrieved April 2, 2010, from http://www.americanheart.org/presenter.jhtml?identifier=4786.

American Thoracic Society. (2002). American Thoracic Society statement: Guidelines for the Six-Minute Walk Test. *American Journal of Respiratory Critical Care Medicine, 166*, 111–117.

Anderson, D.R., Whitmer, R.W., Goetzel, R.Z., Ozminkowski, R.J., Wasserman, J., & Serxner, S.A. (2000, September/October). The relationship between modifiable health risks and group-level health care expenditures: A group-level analysis of the HERO research database. *American Journal of Health Promotion, 15*, 45–52.

Baltes, P.B., & Baltes, M.M. (1990). *Successful aging: Perspectives from the behavioral sciences*. New York: Cambridge University Press.

Bandura, A. (1997). Editorial: The anatomy of stages of changes. *American Journal of Health Promotion, 12*, 8–10.

Baranowski, T., Perry, C.L., & Parcel, G.S. (2002). How individuals, environments, and health behavior interact: Social cognitive theory. In K. Glanz, B.K. Rimer, & F.M. Lewis (Eds.), *Health behavior and health education: Theory, research, and practice* (3rd ed.). San Francisco: Jossey-Bass.

Baur, C. (2007, May). *Health literacy and adults with intellectual and developmental disabilities: Achieving accessible health information and services.* Paper presented at the State of Science in Aging with Developmental Disabilities, Atlanta, Georgia.

Beange, H., McElduff, A., & Baker, W. (1995). Medical disorders of adults with mental retardation: A population study. *American Journal on Mental Retardation, 99*(6), 595–604.

Beck, B.R., & Snow, C.M. (2003). Bone health across the lifespan: Exercising our options. *Exercise and Sport Sciences Reviews, 31*(3), 117–122.

Bell, A.J., & Bhate, M.S. (1992). Prevalence of overweight and obesity in Down syndrome and other mentally handicapped adults living in the community. *Journal of Intellectual Disability Research, 36*(4), 359–364.

Bittles, A.H., Bower, C., Hussain, R., & Glasson, E.J. (2007). The four ages of Down syndrome. *The European Journal of Public Health, 17*(2), 221–225.

Blanck, H.M., Galuska, D.A., Gillespie, C., Kettel-Khan, L., Serdula, M.K., Solera, M.K., et al. (2007). Fruit and vegetable consumption among adults—United States, 2005. *Morbidity and Mortality Weekly Report, 56*(10), 213–217.

Borg, G. (1998). *Borg's Perceived Exertion and Pain Scales.* Champaign, IL: Human Kinetics.

Bohannon, R.W. (1995). Sit-to-stand test for measuring performance of lower extremity muscles. *Perceptual Motor Skills, 80*, 163–166.

Bowe, F.G. (2006). *Video and people with disabilities.* Retrieved April 6, 2007, from http://people.hofstra.edu/faculty/frank_g_bowe/VIDEOindex.html

Braddock, D. (1999). Aging and developmental disabilities: Demographic and policy issues affecting American families. *Mental Retardation, 37*(2), 155–161.

Braddock, D., Hemp, R., & Rizzolo, M.C. (2008). *The state of the states in developmental disabilities* (7th ed.). Washington, DC: American Association on Intellectual and Developmental Disabilities.

Braddock, D., Hemp, R., Rizzolo, M.C., Coulter, D., Haffer, L., & Thompson, M. (2005). *The state of the states in developmental disabilities.* Boulder, CO: University of Colorado, Coleman Institute for Cognitive Disabilities.

Bray, G.A. (1987). Obesity: A disease of nutrient or energy balance? *Nutrition Reviews, 45*, 33–43.p. 129

Burton, W.N., Conti, D.J., Chen, C.Y., Schultz, A.B., & Edington, D.W. (1999). The role of health risk factors and disease on worker productivity. *Journal of Occupational and Environmental Medicine, 41*(10), 863–877.

Canadian Society for Exercise Physiology. (2002*). Physical Activity Readiness Questionnaire (PAR-Q).* Ontario, Canada: Author.

Centers for Disease Control and Prevention. (n.d.). *Behavioral Risk Factor Surveillance System Survey Questionnaire.* Retrieved February 16, 2010, from http://www.cdc.gov/brfs

Centers for Disease Control and Prevention. (2003). *The power of prevention: Reducing the Health and economic burden of chronic disease.* Atlanta, GA: U.S. Department of Health and Human Services. Retrieved March 23, 2010, from http://www.cdc.gov/chronicdisease/overview/pop.htm

Centers for Disease Control and Prevention. (2008a). *Behavioral Risk Factor Surveillance System Survey Data.* Atlanta: U.S. Department of Health and Human Services, Centers for Disease Control and Prevention.

Centers for Disease Control and Prevention. (2008b). *Chronic disease prevention and health promotion: Chronic disease overview.* Retrieved November 18, 2008, from http://www.cdc.gov/nccdphp/overview.htm

Centers for Disease Control and Prevention. (2008c). *Physical activity for everyone.* Retrieved April 28, 2008, from http://www.cdc.gov/nccdphp/dnpa/physical/everyone/index.htm

Centers for Disease Control and Prevention, Division of Nutrition. (2008). *Physical activity and obesity: U.S. physical activity statistics.* Retrieved April 28, 2008, from http://apps.nccd.cdc.gov/PASurveillance/DemoComparev.asp

Chan, J.M., Rimm, E.B., Colditz, G.A., Stampfer, M.J., & Willett, W.C. (1994). Obesity, fat distribution, and weight gain as risk factors for clinical diabetes in men. *Diabetes Care, 17*(9), 961–969.

Colditz, G.A., Willett, W.C., Rotnitzky, A., & Manson, J.E. (1995). Weight gain as a risk factor for clinical diabetes mellitus in women. *Annals of Internal Medicine, 122*(7), 481–486.

College of Education, Wichita State University. (2009). *Handy reminders.* Retrieved September 9, 2009, from http://education.wichita.edu/caduceus/examples/servings/index.htm

Conner, M., & Armitage, C.J. (2002). *The social psychology of food.* Buckingham, UK: Open University Press.

DelParigi, A., Tschöp, M., Heiman, M.L., Salbe, A.D., Vozarova, B., Sell, S.M., et al. (2002). High circulating ghrelin: A potential cause for hyperphagia and obesity in Prader-Willi Syndrome. *The Journal of Clinical Endocrinology and Metabolism, 87*(12), 5461–5464.

Draheim, C.C. (2006). Cardiovascular disease prevalence and risk factors of persons with mental retardation. *Mental Retardation and Developmental Disabilities Research Reviews, 12*(1), 3–12.

Draheim, C.C., McCubbin, J.A., & Williams, D.P. (2002). Differences in cardiovascular disease risk between nondiabetic adults with mental retardation with and without Down syndrome. *American Journal of Mental Retardation, 107*(3), 201–211.

Draheim, C.C., Williams, D.P., & McCubbin, J.A. (2002). Physical activity, dietary intake, and the insulin resistance syndrome in nondiabetic adults with mental retardation. *American Journal of Mental Retardation, 107*(5), 361–375.

Dresser, G.K., Kim, R.B, & Bailey, D.G. (2005). Effects of grapefruit juice volume on the reduction of fexofenading biovaiability: Possible role of organic anion transporting polypeptides. *Clinical Pharmacology & Therapeutics, 77*(3), 170–177.

Drinkwater, B.L.C.H. (1994). McCloy research lecture: Does physical activity play a role in preventing osteoporosis? *Research Quarterly for Exercise and Sport, 65*(3), 197–206.

Eckel, R.H. (1997). Obesity and heart disease: A statement for healthcare professionals from the nutrition committee. *Circulation, 96*, 3248–3250.

Edington, D.W., Yen, L.T., & Witting, P. (1997). The financial impact of changes in personal health practices. *Journal of Occupational and Environmental Medicine, 39*(11), 1037–1047.

Enright, P.L. (2003). The Six-Minute Walk Test. *Respiratory Care, 48*(8), 783–785.

Fielding, J.E. (1990). Worksite health promotion programs in the United States: Progress, lessons, and challenges. *Health Promotion International, 5*(1), 75–84.

Fitzsimons, N. (2000). *Taking charge: Responding to abuse, neglect, and financial exploitation.* Chicago: University of Illinois at Chicago, Department of Disability and Human Development.

Fletcher, G.F., Blair, S.N., Blumenthal, J., et al. (1992). Statement on exercise: Benefits and recommendations for physical activity programs for all Americans. *Circulation, 86*(1), 340–344.

Fox, R.A., Rosenberg, R., & Rotatori, A.F. (1985). Parent involvement in a treatment program for obese retarded adults. *Journal of Behavioral Therapy & Experimental Psychology, 16*, 45–48.

Freeman, S.B., Taft, L.F., Dooley, K.J., Allran, K., Sherman, S.L., Hassold, T.J., et al. (1998). Population-based study of congenital heart defects in Down syndrome. *American Journal of Medical Genetics, 80*(3), 213–217.

Freire, P. (1972). *Pedagogy of the oppressed.* New York: Herder & Herder.

Frey, B., & Rimmer, J.H. (1995). Comparison of body composition between German and American adults with mental retardation. *Medicine and Science in Sports and Exercise, 27*(10), 1439–1443.

Frey, G.C., Buchanan, A.M., & Sandt, D.D.R. (2005). "I'd rather watch TV": An examination of physical activity in adults with mental retardation. *Mental Retardation, 43*(4), 241–254.

Fries, J.F., Harrington, H., Edwards, R., Kent, L.A., & Richardson, N. (1994). Randomized controlled trial of cost reductions from a health education program: The California Public Employees' Retirement System (PERS) study. *American Journal of Health Promotion, 8*(3), 216–223.

Fujiura, G.T. (1998). Demography of family households. *American Journal on Mental Retardation, 103*(3), 225–235.

Fujiura, G.T. (2003). Continuum of intellectual disability: Demographic evidence for the "forgotten generation." *Mental Retardation, 41*(6), 420–429.

Fujiura, G.T., Fitzsimons, N., Marks, B., & Chicoine, B. (1997). Predictors of BMI among adults with Down syndrome: The social context of health promotion. *Research in Developmental Disabilities, 18*(4), 261–274.

Gill, C.J. (1987, Spring). A New Social Perspective on Disability and Its Implications for Rehabilitation, this article appears jointly in *Sociocultural Implications in Treatment Planning in Occupational Therapy* (The Haworth Press, Inc.) and in *Occupational Therapy in Health Care, 7*(1).

Gill, C.J. (1996). Becoming visible: Personal health experiences of women with disabilities. In D.M. Krotoski, M.A. Nosek, & M.A. Turk (Eds.), *Women with physical disabilities: achieving and maintaining health and well-being* (pp. 5–15). Baltimore: Paul H. Brookes Publishing Co.

Gill, C.J. (1997). Four types of integration in disability identity development. *Journal of Vocational Rehabilitation, 9*(1), 39–46.

Glasgow, R.E., McCaul, K.D., & Fisher, K.J. (1993). Participation in worksite health promotion: A critique of the literature and recommendations for future practice. *Health Education & Behavior, 20*(3), 391–408.

Glasgow, R.E., & Terborg, J.R. (1988). Occupational health promotion programs to reduce cardiovascular risk. *Journal of Consulting and Clinical Psychology, 56*(3), 365–373.

Goetzel, R.Z., Anderson, D.R., Whitmer, R.W., Ozminkowski, R.J., Dunn, R.L., & Wasserman J. (1998). Health Enhancement Research Organization (HERO) Research Committee. The relationship between modifiable health risks and health care expenditures: An analysis of the multiemployer HERO health risk and cost database. *Journal of Occupational and Environmental Medicine, 40*(10), 843–854.

Goetzel, R.Z., Juday, T.R., & Ozminkowski, R.J. (1999, Summer). "What's the ROI?" a systematic review of return on investment (ROI) studies of corporate health and productivity management initiatives. *AWHP's Worksite Health, 6,* 12–21.

Gold, D.B., Anderson, D.A., & Serxner, S. (2000, Nov/Dec). Impact of a telephone-based intervention on the reduction of health risks. *American Journal of Health Promotion 15*(2), 97–106.

Gottschalk, J. (1999). Nursing and sustainable development. *Nursing in the Americas, 571.* Washington, DC: Pan American Health Organization.

Granger, C.V., Mann, W.C., Ottenbacher, K.J., Tomita, M.R., & Fiedler, R.C. (1994). Functional measures of geriatric subjects in the community. *Topics in Geriatric Rehabilitation, 10*(1), 7–21.

Grantmakers Health. (2004). Healthy behaviors: addressing chronic disease at its roots. *Issue Brief, 2*(19), 1–39.

Gross, M.M., Stevenson, P.J., Charette, S.L., Pyka, G., & Marcus, R. (1998). Effect of muscle strength and movement speed on the biomechanics of rising from a chair in healthy elderly and young women. *Gait Posture, 8*(3), 175–85.

Grundy, S.M., Bazzarre, T., Cleeman, J., et al. (2000). Prevention conference V: Beyond secondary prevention: Identifying the high-risk patient for primary prevention; medical office assessment. *Circulation, 101*(1), e3–e11.

Gurwitz, J.H., & Avorn, J.(1991). The ambiguous relationship between aging and adverse drug reactions. *Annals of Internal Medicine, 114*(11), 956–966.

Haffner, S., & Taegtmeyer, H. (2003). Epidemic obesity and the metabolic syndrome. *Circulation, 108*(13), 1541–1545.

Halperin, J.A. (1998). Setting health standards for the 21st century. *Journal of the American Pharmaceutical Association, 38*(6), 762–766.

Harris, N., Rosenberg, A., Jangda, S., O'Brien, K., & Gallagher, M. (2003). Prevalence of obesity in International Special Olympic athletes as determined by body mass index. *Journal of the American Dietetic Association, 103*(2), 235–237.

Haveman, M. (2007, May). *Health indicators for adults with intellectual disabilities in Europe.* Paper presented at the State of Science in Aging with Developmental Disabilities. Rehabilitation Research and Training Center on Aging with Developmental Disabilities, Atlanta, GA.

Hawkings, B.A., Ardovino, P., & Hsieh, C. (1998). Validity and reliability of the Leisure Assessment Inventory. *Mental Retardation, 36*(4), 303–313.

Hayden, M.F. (1998). Mortality among people with mental retardation living in the United States: Research review and policy application. *Mental Retardation, 36*, 345–359.

Hedley, A.A., Ogden, C.L., Johnson, C.L., Carroll, M.D., Curtin, L.R., & Flegal, K. (2004). Overweight and obesity among U.S. children, adolescents, and adults: 1999–2002. *Journal of the American Medical Association, 291*, 2847–2850.

Heller, T. (2001a). Self-efficacy scale. In T. Heller, B.A. Marks, & S.H. Ailey (Eds.), *Exercise and nutrition education curriculum for adults with developmental disabilities* (p. A.12). Rehabilitation Research and Training Center on Aging and Developmental Disabilities, University of Illinois at Chicago.

Heller, T. (2001b). Social/Environmental Supports Scale. In T. Heller, B.A. Marks, & S.H. Ailey *Exercise and nutrition education curriculum for adults with developmental disabilities.* Rehabilitation Research and Training Center on Aging and Developmental Disabilities. Department of Disability and Human Development, University of Illinois at Chicago.

Heller, T., Hsieh, K., & Rimmer, J. (2000, November). *Exercise adherence among older adults with mental retardation: Exercise knowledge, fitness, and life satisfaction outcomes.* Paper presentation at the Gerontological Society of America Annual Meeting, Washington, DC.

Heller, T., Hsieh, K., & Rimmer, J.H. (2004). Attitudinal and psychological outcomes of a fitness and health education program on adults with Down syndrome. *American Journal on Mental Retardation, 109*(2), 175–185.

Heller, T., & Marks, B. (2002). Health promotion and women. In P.N. Walsh & T. Heller (Eds.), *Health promotion and women with intellectual disabilities* (pp. 170–189). London: Blackwell Science Publishing.

Heller, T., Marks, B., & Ailey, S. (2001). *Exercise and nutrition health education curriculum for adults with developmental disabilities.* Chicago: University of Illinois Rehabilitation Research and Training Center on Aging with Developmental Disabilities.

Heller, T., Marks, B., Pastorfield, C., Sisirak, J., & Hsieh, K. (2006, November). *Outcomes of five community-based health promotion programs across the U.S. for athletes with intellectual disabilities,* American Public Health Association, 134th Annual Meeting and Exposition, Boston, MA.

Heller, T., Miller, A., Hsieh, K., & Sterns, H. (2000). Later life planning: Promoting knowledge of options and choice-making. *Mental Retardation, 38*(5), 395–406.

Heller, T., & Prochaska, T.J. (2001). Exercise perception scale. In T. Heller, B.A. Marks, & S.H. Ailey (Eds.), *Exercise and nutrition education curriculum for adults with developmental disabilities* (p. A.9). Chicago: Rehabilitation Research and Training Center on Aging and Developmental Disabilities, University of Illinois at Chicago.

Heller, T., Rimmer, J., & Rubin, S. (2001). Barriers scale. In T. Heller, B.A. Marks, & S.H. Ailey (Eds.), Exercise and nutrition education curriculum for adults with developmental disabilities (pp. A.9–A.10). Chicago: Rehabilitation Research and Training Center on Aging and Developmental Disabilities.

Heller, T., Sterns, H., Sutton, E., & Factor, A. (1996). Impact of person-centered later life planning training program for older adults with mental retardation. *Journal of Rehabilitation, 62*(5), 77–83.

Heller, T., Ying, H.S., Rimmer, J.H., & Marks, B.A. (2002). Determinants of exercise in adults with cerebral palsy. *Public Health Nursing, 19*(3), 223–231.

Heyward, V.H. (2006). Advanced fitness assessment and exercise prescription (5th ed., p. 254). Champagne, IL: Human Kinetics.

Hollins, S., Downer, J., Perez, W., et al. (2000). Screening women for breast and cervical cancer. *Journal of Intellectual Disability Research, 44*, 322–323.

Hollins, S., & Perez, W. (2000). *Looking at my breasts.* London: Royal College of Psychiatry.

Holm, V.A., Cassidy, S.B., Butler, M.G., Hancett, J.M., Greenswag, L.R., Whitman, B.Y., et al. (1993). Prader-Willi syndrome: Consensus diagnostic criteria. *Pediatrics, 91*, 398–402.

Hornsten, A., Sandstrom, H., & Lundman, B. (2004). Personal understandings of illness among people with Type 2 diabetes. *Journal of Advanced Nursing, 47*(2), 174–182.

Hsieh, K., Heller, T., & Miller, A.B. (2001). Risk factors for injuries and falls among adults with developmental disabilities. *Journal of Intellectual Disability Research, 45*(1), 76–82.

Hu, F.B., Li, T.Y., Colditz, G., Willett, W.C., & Manson, J.E. (2003). Television watching and other sedentary behaviors in relation to risk of obesity and Type 2 Diabetes Mellitus in women. *Journal of the American Medical Association, 289*(14), 1785–1791.

Hubert, H.B., Feinleib, M., McNamara, P.M., & Castelli, W.P. (1983). Obesity as an independent risk factor for cardiovascular disease: A 26-year follow-up of participants in the Framingham Heart Study. *Circulation, 67*(5), 968–977.

Hui, S.S., & Yuen, P.Y. (2000). Validity of the modified back-saver sit-and-reach test: A comparison with other protocols. *Medicine & Science in Sports & Exercise, 32*(9), 1655–1659.

Iacono, T., & Sutherland, G. (2006). Health screening and developmental disabilities. *Journal of Policy and Practice in Intellectual Disabilities, 3*(3), 155–163.

Illingworth, K., Moore, K.A., & McGillivray, J. (2003). The development of the nutrition and activity knowledge scale for use with people with an intellectual disability. *Journal of Applied Research in Intellectual Disabilities, 16*, 159–66.

Institute of Medicine Committee on Health Care in America. (2001). *Crossing the quality chasm: A new health system for the 21st century.* Washington, DC: National Academies Press.

Issel, M.L. (2004). *Health promotion planning and evaluation: A practical, systemic approach for community health.* Sudbury, MA: Jones & Bartlett Publishers.

Janicki, M., Dalton, A., Henderson, C., & Davidson, P. (1999). Mortality and morbidity among older adults with intellectual disability: Health service considerations. *Disability & Rehabilitation, 21*, 284–294.

Janicki, M., Davidson, P., Henderson, C., McCallion, P., Taets, J., & Force, L. (2002). Health characteristics and health services utilization in older adults with intellectual disability living in community residences. *Journal of Intellectual Disability Research, 46*(4), 287–298.

Jansen, D.E.M.C., Krol, B., Groothoff, J.W., & Post, D. (2004). People with intellectual disability and their health problems: A review of comparative studies. *Journal of Intellectual Disability Research, 48*(2), 93–102.

Johnson, T.F. (1995). Aging well in contemporary society: Introduction. *American Behavioral Scientist, 39*(2), 120–130.

Kalnins, I., McQueen, D.V., Backett, K.C., Curtice, L., & Currie, C.E. (1992). Children, empowerment, and health promotion: Some new directions in research and practice. *Health Promotion International, 7*, 53–59.

Kervio, G., Carre, F., & Ville, N. (2003). Reliability and intensity of the six-minute walk test in healthy elderly subjects. *Medicine & Science in Sports & Exercise, 35*(1), 169–174.

Knivsberg, A.M., Reichelt, K.L, Holden, T., & Nodland, M. (2002). A randomized, controlled study of dietary intervention in autistic syndromes. *Nutritional Neuroscience, 5*(4), 251–261.

Knivsberg, A.M., Reichelt, K.L., & Nodland, M. (2001) Reports on dietary intervention in autistic disorders. *Nutritional Neuroscience, 4*(1), 25–37.

Kopac, C.A., Fritz, J., & Holt, R. (1996). *Availability and accessibility of gynecological and reproductive services for women with developmental disabilities.* Washington, DC: American Network of Community Options and Resources.

Kovacs, M. (1985). The Children's Depression Inventory. *Psychopharmacology Bulletin, 21*, 995–998.

Krain, M.A. (1995). Policy implications for a society aging well: Employment, retirement, education, and leisure policies for the 21st century. *American Behavioral Scientist, 39*(2), 131–151.

Laffrey, S.C. (1985). Health behavior choice as related to self-actualization and health conception. *Western Journal of Nursing Research, 7*(3), 279–295.

Laffrey, S.C. (1986). Development of a health conception scale. *Research in Nursing and Health, 9*, 107–113.

Laforge, R.G., Greene, G.W., & Procohaska, J.O. [1994]. Psycho-social factors influencing low fruit and vegetable consumption. *Journal of Behavioral Medicine, 17*, 361–374.

Laforge, R.G., Velicer, W.F., Richmond, R.L., & Owen, N. (1999). Stage distributions for five health behaviors in the USA and Australia. *Prevention Medicine, 28*, 61–74.

Larson, S.A., Lakin, K.C., Anderson, L., Kwak, N., Lee, J.H., & Anderson, D. (2001). Prevalence of mental retardation and developmental disabilities: Estimates from the 1994/1995 National Health Interview Survey Disability Supplements. *American Journal of Mental Retardation, 106*(3), 231–252.

Lawton, M.P., Moss, M., Fulcomer, M., & Kleban, M.H. (1982). A research and service oriented multilevel assessment instrument. *Journal of Gerontology, 37*, 91–99.

Lennox, N.G., Diggens, J.N., & Ugoni, A.M. (1997). The general practice care of people with intellectual disability: Barriers and solutions. *Journal of Intellectual Disability Research 41*(5), 380–390.

Lewis, M.A., Lewis, C.E., Leake, B., King, B.H., & Lindemann, R. (2002). The quality of health care for adults with developmental disabilities. *Public Health Report, 117*(2), 174–184.

Linton, S. (1998). *Claiming disability: Knowledge and identity.* New York: New York University Press.

Loehr, J.P., Synhorst, D.P., Wolfe, R.R., et al. (1986). Aortic root dilatation and mitral valve prolapse in fragile X syndrome. *American Journal of Medical Genetics, 23*, 189–194.

Lorig, K., Brown, B.W. Jr., Ung, E., Chastain, R., Shoor, S., & Holman, H.R. (1989). Development and evaluation of a scale to measure the perceived self-efficacy of people with arthritis. *Arthritis and Rheumatism, 32*(1), 37–44.

Lorig K., Stewart, A., Ritter, P., González, V., Laurent, D., & Lynch, J. (1996). *Outcome measures for health education and other health care interventions.* Thousand Oaks, CA: Sage Publications, 52–53.

Lucas, B.L., & Byler, E. (2003). Postion of the American Dietetic Association: Nutrition in comprehensive program planning for persons with developmental disabilities. *Journal of the American Dietetic Association, 97*(2), 189–193.

Lunsky, Y., & Havercamp, S.M. (2002). Women's mental health. In P.N. Walsh & T. Heller (Eds.), *Health of women with intellectual disabilities* (pp. 170–189). Oxford: Blackwell Science Publishing.

Lynch, J.W., Smith, G.D., Kaplan, G.A., et al. (2000). Income inequality and mortality: Importance to health of individual income, psychosocial environment, and material conditions. *British Medical Journal, 320*, 1200–1204.

Mann, J., Zhou, H., McDermott, S., & Poston, M.B. (2006). Healthy behavior change of adults with mental retardation: Attendance in a health promotion program. *American Journal on Mental Retardation, 3*(1), 62–73.

Marks, B. (1996). *Conceptualizations of health among adults with intellectual impairments,* Unpublished doctoral dissertation, University of Illinois at Chicago.

Marks, B., & Heller, T. (2003). Bridging the equity gap: Health promotion for adults with developmental disabilities. *Nursing Clinics of North America, 38*(2), 205–228.

Marks, B., Heller, T., Sisirak, J., Hsieh, K., & Pastorfield, C. (2005). *Health promotion pilot programs evaluation: Improving athletes' health: Final report.* Washington, DC: Special Olympics International.

Marks, B., Sisirak, J., & Donahue Chase, D. (2008). *Pilot testing of a Health Promotion Capacity Checklist for community-based organizations.* Paper presented at the IASSID 13th World Congress, People with Intellectual Disabilities: Citizens of the World.

Marks, B., Sisirak, J., & Heller, T. (2008, August 29). *Efficacy of a Train-the-Trainer Program on caregivers' health status, perceptions, and behavior.* Paper presented at IASSID 13th World Congress, People with Intellectual Disabilities: Citizens of the World, Cape Town, South Africa.

Marks, B., Sisirak, J., & Heller, T. (2010). *Health matters: The exercise and nutrition health education curriculum for people with developmental disabilities.* Baltimore: Paul H. Brookes Publishing Co.

Marks, B., Sisirak, J., Heller, T., & Hsieh, K. (2005, December). *Health status, perceptions, and behavior of staff working with people with intellectual and developmental disabilities*, Paper presented at the meeting of the American Public Health Association, 133rd Annual Meeting and Exposition, Philadelphia.

Marks, B., Sisirak, J., Heller, T., & Riley, B. (2006, November). *Efficacy of a train-the-trainer program to improve health status for people with intellectual and developmental disabilities*. Paper presented at the meeting of the American Public Health Association, 134th Annual Meeting and Exposition, Boston.

Marks, B., Sisirak, J., Heller, T., & Riley, B. (2007, November). *Impact of a train-the-trainer program on the psychosocial health status of staff supporting adults with intellectual and developmental disabilities*. Paper presented at the meeting of the American Public Health Association, 135th Annual Meeting and Exposition, Washington, DC.

Marks, B., Sisirak, J., & Hsieh, K. (2008). Health services, health promotion, and health literacy: Report from the State of the Science in Aging with Developmental Disabilities Conference. *Disability and Health Journal, 1*(3), 136–142.

Mayo Clinic. (n.d.). Diabetes and exercise: When to monitor your blood sugar. Retrieved September 9, 2009, at http://www.mayoclinic.com/health/diabetes-and-exercise/DA00105

McCarron, M., Gill, M., McCallion, P., & Begley, C. (2005). Health co-morbidities in aging persons with Down syndrome and Alzheimer's dementia. *Journal of Intellectual Disability Research, 49*(7), 560–566.

McDaniel, J.H., Hunt, A., Hackes, B., & Pope, J.F. (2001). Impact of dining room environment on nutritional intake of Alzheimer's disease: A pilot study. *American Journal of Alzheimer's Disease, 10*(6), 40–44.

McKnight, J. (1995). *Careless society: Community and its counterfeits.* New York: Basic Books.

McLeroy, K.R., Bibeau, D., Steckler, A. & Glanz, K. (1988). An ecological perspective on health promotion programs. *Health Education & Behavior 15*(4), 351–377.

McNamara, C. (2008). *Basic guide to program evaluation.* Retrieved November 18, 2008, from http://www.mapnp.org/library/evaluatn/fnl_eval.htm

Medlen, J.E.G. (2002). *The Down syndrome nutrition handbook: A guide to promoting healthy lifestyles.* Bethesda, MD: Woodbine House.

Melville, C.A., Cooper, S.A., McGrother, C.W., Thorp, C.F., & Collacott, R. (2005). Obesity in adults with Down syndrome: A case–control study. *Journal of Intellectual Disability Research, 49*(2), 125–133.

Melville, C.A., Finlayson, J., Cooper, S.A., Allan, L., Robinson, N., Burns, E., et al. (2005). Enhancing primary health care services for adults with intellectual disabilities. *Journal of Intellectual Disability Research, 49*(3), 190–198.

Melville, C.A., Hamilton, S., Hankey, C.R., Miller, S., & Boyle, S. (2006). The prevalence and determinants of obesity in adults with intellectual disabilities. *Obesity Reviews, 8*(3), 223–230. Retrieved March 20, 2007, from http://www.blackwell-synergy.com/doi/full/10.1111/j.1467789X.2006.00296.x?prevSearch=allfield%3A%28The+prevalence+and+determinants+of+obesity+in+adults+with+intellectual+disabilities%29

Messent, P.R., Cooke, C.B., & Long, J. (1999). What choice? A consideration of the level of opportunity for people with mild and moderate learning disabilities to lead a physically active healthy lifestyle. *British Journal of Learning Disabilities, 27*, 73–77.

Messias, D.K., Hall, J.M., & Meleis, A.I. (1996). Voices of impoverished Brazilian women: Health implications of roles and resources. *Woman & Health, 24*(1), 1–20.

Miotto, J.M., Chodzko-Zajko, W.J., Reich, J.L., & Supler, M.M. (1999). Reliability and validity of the Fullerton Functional Fitness Test: An independent replication study. *Journal of Aging and Physical Activity, 7*, 339–353.

Miziniak, H. (1994). Persons with Alzheimer's: Effects of nutrition and exercise. *Journal of Gerontological Nursing, 20*(10), 27–32.

Morse, J.S., & Roth, S.P. (1994). Sexuality. In S.P. Roth & J.S. Morse (Eds.), *A life-span approach to nursing care for individuals with developmental disabilities* (pp. 281–295). Baltimore: Paul H. Brookes Publishing Co.

Mullen, P.D. (1988). Health promotion and patient education benefits for employees. *Annual Review of Public Health, 9*, 305–332.

Must, A., Spadano, J., Coakley, E.H., Field, A.E., Colditz, G., & Dietz, W.H. (1999). The disease burden associated with overweight and obesity. *Journal of the American Medical Association, 282*(16), 1523–1529.

National Center for Chronic Disease Prevention and Health Promotion. (2007). Behavioral Risk Factor Surveillance System: Weight classification by Body Mass Index (BMI). Retrieved March 23, 2010, from http://apps.nccd.cdc.gov/gisbrfss/map.aspx

National Center for Education Statistics. (2003). *National assessment of Adult Literacy Institute of Education Sciences.* Washington, DC: U.S. Department of Education.

National Center for Health Statistics. (1995). Report of final mortality statistics. *Monthly Vital Statistics Report, 45*(11), Supplement 2, 1–80.

National Heart, Lung, and Blood Institute. (2010). Guide to physical activity. Retrieved March 1, 2010, from http://www.nhlbi.nih.gov/health/public/heart/obesity/lose_wt/phy_act.htm

National Heart, Lung, and Blood Institute's Obesity Education Initiative. (1995). Clinical guidelines on the identification, evaluation, and treatment of obesity in adults: Executive summary. *American Journal of Clinical Nutrition, 68*, 899–917.

National Institute of Diabetes and Digestive and Kidney Diseases. http://diabetes.niddk.nih.gov/dm/pubs/physical_ez/index.htm

National Institute of Diabetes and Digestive Kidney Diseases. (2007). *Obesity, physical activity, and weight-control glossary.* Retrieved May 4, 2007, from http://win.niddk.nih.gov/publications/glossary.htm

National Institutes of Health. (2006). In brief: Your guide to lowering your blood pressure with DASH. Retrieved March 1, 2010, from http://www.nhlbi.nih.gov/health/public/heart/hbp/dash/dash_inbrief.htm

National Institutes of Health. (2009). *Detailed budget for initial budget period.* Retrieved January 2, 2010, from http://www.grants.nih.gov/grants/funding/phs398/fp4.doc

National Organization on Disability. (1998). *NOD/Harris Survey of Americans with Disabilities.* Washington, DC: The National Organization on Disability.

National Osteoporosis Foundation. (n.d.). Prevention: Exercise for Health Bones. Retrieved March 1, 2010, from http://www.nof.org/prevention/exercise.htm

National Task Force on the Prevention and Treatment of Obesity. (2000). Overweight, obesity, and health risk. *Archives of Internal Medicine, 160*(7), 898–904.

Nestle, M., Wing, R., Birch, L., DiSogra, L., Drewnowski, A., Middleton, S., et al. (1998). Behavioral and social influences on food choice. *Nutrition Reviews, 56*(5), S50–S64.

Newby, P.K., Muller, D., Hallfrisch, J., Qiao, N., Andres, R., & Tucker, K.L. (2003). Dietary patterns and changes in body mass index and waist circumference in adults. *American Journal of Clinical Nutrition, 77*(6), 1417–1425.

Nigg, C., Hellsten, L., Norman, G., Braun, L., Breger, R., Burbank, P., et al. (2005). Physical activity staging distribution: Establishing a heuristic using multiple studies. *Annals of Behavioral Medicine, 29*(2), 35–45.

Nirje, B. (1969). The normalization principle and its human management implications. In R. Kugel & W. Wolfensberger (Eds.), *Changing patterns in residential services for the mentally retarded.* Washington, DC: President's Committee on Mental Retardation.

O'Brien, C.L., O'Brien, J., & Mount, B. (1997). Person-centered planning has arrived … or has it? *Mental Retardation, 35*(6), 480–484.

O'Brien, D.R. (1994). Health maintenance and promotion in adults. In S.P. Roth & J.S. Morse (Eds.), *A life-span approach to nursing care for individuals with developmental disabilities* (pp. 171–192). Baltimore: Paul H. Brookes Publishing Co.

O'Donnell, M.P., & Ainsworth, T.H. (Eds.). (1984). *Health promotion in the workplace.* New York: Wiley.

Ogden, C.L., Carroll, M.D., Curtin, L.R., McDowell, M.A., Tabak, C.J., & Flegal, K.M. (2006). Prevalence of overweight and obesity in the United States, 1999–2004. *Journal of the American Medical Association, 295,* 1549–1555.

Oh-Park, M., Zohman, L.R., & Abrahams, C. (1997). A simple walk test to guide exercise programming of the elderly. *American Journal of Physical Medicine and Rehabilitation, 76*(3), 208–212.

O'Keefe, S.T., Lye, M., Donnellan, C., & Carmichael, D.N. (1998). Reproducibility and responsiveness of quality of life assessment and six minute walk test in elderly heart failure patients. *Heart, 80*(4), 377–382.

O'Malley, A.S., Kerner, J.F., & Johnson, L. (1999). Are we getting the message out to all? Health information sources and ethnicity. *American Journal of Preventative Medicine, 17*(3), 198–202.

Palmer, C.A. (2001). Important relationships between diet, nutrition, and oral health. *Nutrition Clinical Care, 4*(1), 5–14.

Pan American Health Organization. (2001). *Promoting health in the Americas annual report of the director.* Washington, DC: World Health Organization.

Pan American Health Organization. (2002). *Strategic and programmatic orientations, 1999–2002,* Document # 291. Washington, DC: Pan American Sanitary Bureau.

Patja, K., Iivanainen, M., Vesala, H., Oksanen, H., & Ruoppila, I. (2000). Life expectancy of people with intellectual disability: A 35-year follow-up study. *Journal of Intellectual Disability Research, 44*(5), 591–599.

Pelletier, K.R. (1999). A review and analysis of the clinical and cost-effectiveness studies of comprehensive health promotion and disease management programs at the worksite: 1995–1998 update (IV). *American Journal of Health Promotion, 13*(6), 333–345.

Pender, N.J. (1987). *Health promotion in nursing practice* (5th ed.). Norwalk, CT: Appleton & Lange.

Phillips, A., Morrison, J., & Davis, R.W. (2004). General practitioners' educational needs in intellectual disability health. *Journal of Intellectual Disability Research, 48*(2).

Pi-Sunyer, F.X. (1999). Comorbidities of overweight and obesity: current evidence and research issues. Medicine & Science in Sports & Exercise, 31(11 Suppl), S602–608.

Podsiadlo, D., & Richardson, S. (1991). The timed 'up and go' test: A test of basic functional mobility for frail elderly persons. *Journal of American Geriatric Society, 39,* 142–148.

Prasher, V.P. (1995). Overweight and obesity amongst Down syndrome adults. *Journal of Intellectual Disability Research, 39*(5), 437–441.

Prasher, V.P., & Janicki, M.P. (2002). *Physical health of adults with intellectual disabilities.* Oxford, UK: Blackwell Publishing.

Prochaska, J.M., Prochaska, J.O., & Levesque, D.A. (2001). A transtheoretical approach to changing organizations. *Administration and Policy in Mental Health, 28*(4), 247–261.

Prochaska, J.O., & DiClemente, C.C. (1983). Stages and processes of self-change of smoking: Toward an integrative model of change. *Journal of Consulting and Clinical Psychology, 51,* 390–395.

Prochaska, J.O., & DiClemente, C.C. (1992). Stages of change in the modification of problem behaviors. In M. Hersen, R. Eisler, & P. Miller (Eds.), *Progress in Behavior Modification 28,* 183–218.

Prochaska, J.O., DiClemente, C.C., & Norcross, J.C. (1992). In search of how people change: Applications to addictive behavior. *American Psychologist, 47,* 1102–1114.

Prochaska, J.O., Velicer, W.F., Rossie, J.S., Goldstein, M.G., Marcus, B.H., Rakowski, W., et al. (1994). Stages of change and decisional balance for 12 problem behaviors. *Health Psychology, 13,* 38–46.

Prouty, R.W., Smith, G., & Lakin, K.C. (2006). *Residential services for persons with developmental disabilities: Status and trends through 2005.* Minneapolis: University of Minnesota Research and Training Center on Community Living.

Rikli, R.E., & Jones, C.J. (1999). Development and validation of a functional fitness test for community-residing older adults. *Journal of Aging and Physical Activity, 7*, 129–161.

Rimmer, J.H., Braddock, D., & Fujiura, G.T. (1993). Prevalence of obesity in adults with mental retardation: Implications for health promotion and disease prevention. *Mental Retardation, 31*(2), 105–110.

Rimmer, J.H., Braddock, D., & Fujiura, G.T. (1994). Cardiovascular risk factor levels in adults with mental retardation. *American Journal of Mental Retardation, 98*(4), 510–518.

Rimmer, J.H., Braddock, D., & Marks, B.A. (1995). Health characteristics and behaviors of adults with mental retardation residing in three living arrangements. *Research in Developmental Disabilities, 16*(6), 489–499.

Rimmer, J.H., & Rubin, S.S. (1996, August). *Exercise, health, activity patterns, and barriers to exercise in adults with physical disabilities.* Paper presented at the NIH Paralympic Congress Proceedings, Atlanta.

Rimmer, J.H., & Wang, E. (2005). Obesity prevalence among a group of Chicago residents with disabilities. *Archives of Physical Medicine and Rehabiliation, 86*(7), 1461–1464.

Rimmer, J.H., & Yamaki, K. (2006). Obesity and intellectual disability. *Mental Retardation & Developmental Disabilities Research Reviews, 12*(1), 22–27.

Robertson, J., Emerson, E., Gregory, N., Hatton, C., Turner, S., Kessissoglou, S., et al. (2000). Lifestyle related risk factors for poor health in residential settings for people with intellectual disabilities. *Research in Developmental Disabilities, 21*(6), 469–486.

Rodgers, J. (1998). "Whatever's on her plate": Food in the lives of people with learning disabilities. *British Journal of Learning Disabilities, 26*, 13–26.

Rolls, B.J., Morris, E.L., & Roe, L.S. (2002). Portion size of food affects energy intake in normal-weight and overweight men and women. *American Journal of Clinical Nutrition, 76*(6), 1207–1213.

Rubin, S.S., Rimmer, J.H., Chicoine, B., Braddock, D., & McGuire, D. (1998). Overweight prevalence in persons with Down syndrome. *Mental Retardation, 36*(3), 175–181.

Ryan, C., Kline, M., Hamrick, D., & Edwards, K. (1995). Caregivers and the nutritional needs of the patient with Alzheimer's disease: A pilot study. *American Journal of Alzheimer's Disease, 10*(6), 40–44.

Sallis, J.F., Grossman, R.M., Pinski, R.B., Patterson, T.L., & Nader, P.R. (1987). The development of scales to measure social support for diet and exercise behaviors. *Preventive Medicine, 16*, 825–836.

Scheerenberger, R. (1987). *A history of mental retardation: A quarter century of promise.* Baltimore: Paul H. Brookes Publishing Co.

Schein, E.H. (1990). Organization culture. *American Psychologist, 45*(2), 109–119.

Selden, C.R., Zorn, M., Ratzan, S., & Parker, R.M. (2000). *Health literacy: January 1990 through October 1999.* Bethesda, MD: National Library of Medicine.

Serxner, S.A., Gold, D.B., Anderson, D.R., & Williams, D. (2001). The impact of a worksite health promotion program on short-term disability usage. *Journal of Occupational and Environmental Medicine, 43*(1), 25–29.

Shankar, S., & Klassen, A. (2001). Influence on fruit and vegetable procurement and consumption among urban African American public housing residents and potential strategies for intervention. *Family Economics and Nutrition Review, 13*(2), 34–46.

Sisirak, J., Marks, B., & Heller, T. (2005, December). *Reliability of Adapted Nutrition and Activity Knowledge Scale for people with intellectual disabilities.* Paper presented at American Public Health Association, 133rd Annual Meeting & Exposition, Philadelphia.

Sisirak, J., Marks, B., Heller, T., & Riley, B. (2007, November). *Dietary habits of adults with intellectual and developmental disabilities residing in community-based settings.* Paper presented at the American Public Health Association, 135th Annual Meeting and Exposition, Washington, DC.

Sisirak, J., Marks, B., Riley, B., & Chang, Y.C. (2008, October). *Patterns of medication use and health status among adults with I/DD.* Paper presented at the American Public Health Association, 136th Annual Meeting & Exposition, San Diego, CA.

Sisirak, J., Marks, B., Riley, B., & Heller, T. (2008, August). *Factors associated with fruit and vegetable intake among adults with I/DD.* Paper presented at the IASSID 13th World Congress, People with Intellectual Disabilities: Citizens of the World, Cape Town, South Africa.

Stewart, D.E. (1992). High-fiber diet and serum tricyclic antidepressant. *Journal of Clinical Psychopharmacology, 12*(6), 438–440.

Sturm, R., & Wells, K.B. (2001). Does obesity contribute as much to morbidity as poverty or smoking? *Public Health Nursing, 115*, 229–235.

Tarlov, A.R. (1996). Social determinants of health: The sociobiological translation. In D. Blane, E. Brunner, & R. Wilkinson (Eds.), Health and social organization: Towards a health policy for the twenty-first century (pp. 71). New York: Routledge, Taylor & Francis.

Turk, V., & Burchell, S. (2003). Developing and evaluating personal health records for adults with learning disabilities. *Tizard Learning Disability Review, 8*(4), 33–41.

U.S. Coast Guard. (2001). *Designing your program workbook: Coast guard health promotion.* Retrieved February 16, 2010, from http://www.uscg.mil/WORKLIFE

U.S. Department of Agriculture. (2003). *Agriculture fact book 2001–2002.* Retrieved November 18, 2008, from http://www.usda.gov/factbook/2002factbook.pdf

U.S. Department of Agriculture. (2005). *Dietary Guidelines for Americans 2005.* Retrieved March 25, 2010, from http://www.health.gov/dietaryguidelines/dga2005/recommendations.htm

U.S. Department of Agriculture, Center for Nutrition Policy and Promotion. (2005). Anatomy of MyPyramid. Retrieved January 2, 2010, from http://www.mypyramid.gov/downloads/MyPyramid_Anatomy.pdf

U.S. Department of Health and Human Services. (2000). *Healthy people 2010: With understanding and improving health and objectives for improving health* (2nd ed., Vols. 1–2). Washington, DC: U.S. Government Printing Office.

U.S. Department of Health and Human Services. (2001). *The Surgeon General's call to action to prevent and decrease overweight and obesity.* Retrieved March 22, 2007, from http://www.surgeongeneral.gov/sgoffice.htm

U.S. Department of Health and Human Services. (2005a). *Dietary Guidelines for Americans 2005.* Retrieved February 2, 2010, from http://www.health.gov/dietaryguidelines/

U.S. Department of Health and Human Services. (2005b). *The Surgeon General's call to action to improve the health and wellness of persons with disabilities.* Rockville: Author.

U.S. Public Health Service. (2002). *Closing the gap: A national blueprint for improving the health of individuals with mental retardation.* Report of the Surgeon General's Conference on Health Disparities and Mental Retardation. Washington, DC: Author.

van Schrojenstein, H.M., & Valk, L.D. (2005). Health in people with intellectual disabilities: Current knowledge and gaps in knowledge. *Journal of Applied Research in Intellectual Disabilities, 18*(4), 325–333.

Velicer, W.F., Fava, J.L., Prochaska, J.O., Abrams, D.B., Emmore, K.M., & Pierce, J.P. (1995). Distribution of smokers by stage in three representative samples. *Preventive Medicine, 24*, 401–411.

Vignehsa, H., Soh, G., Lo, G.L., et al. (1991). Dental health of disabled children in Singapore. *Australian Dental Journal, 36*(2), 151–156.

Wall, J.C., Bell, C., Campbell, S., & Davis, J. (2000). The Timed Get-up-and-Go Test revisited: Measurement of the component tasks. *Journal of Rehabilitation Research & Development, 37*(1), 109–13.

Wallace, E. (2005). Television and nutrition in juvenile detention centers. *Californian Journal of Health Promotion, 3*(2), 125–129.

Walsh, P.N. (2002). Women's health: A contextual approach. In P.N. Walsh & T. Heller (Eds.), *Health promotion and women with intellectual disabilities* (pp. 7–21). London: Blackwell Publishing.

Wardlaw, G.M., Insel, P.M., & Seyler, M.F. (1994). *Contemporary nutrition: Issues and insights.* St. Louis: Mosby.

Ware, J.E., & Sherbourne, C.D. (1992). The MOS 36-Item Short Form Health Survey (SF-36): Conceptual framework and item selection. *Medical Care, 30*(6), 473–483.

Warner, K.E., Wickizer, T.M., Wolfe, R.A., Schildroth, J.E., & Samuelson, M.H. (1988). Economic implications of workplace health promotion programs: Review of the literature. *Journal of Occupational Medicine, 30,* 106–112.

Welling, P.G. (1996). Effects of food on drug absorption. *Annual Review of Nutrition, 16,* 383–415.

White-Scott, S. (2007, May). *Health care and health promotion for aging individuals with intellectual diabilities.* Paper presented at the State of Science in Aging with Developmental Disabilities, Atlanta.

Winett, R.A., King, A.C., & Altman, D.G. (1989). *Health psychology and public health: An integrative approach.* New York: Pergamon Press.

Wolff, I., van Croonenborg, J.J., Kemper, H.C.G., Kostense, P.J. & Twisk, J.W.R. (1999). The Effect of exercise training programs on bone mass: A meta-analysis of published controlled trials in pre- and postmenopausal women. *Osteoporosis International, 9*(1), 1–12.

Wood, E.A., Olmstead, G.W., & Craig, J.L. (1989). An evaluation of lifestyle risk factors and absenteeism after two years in a worksite health promotion programs. *American Journal of Health Promotion, 4*(2), 128–113.

World Health Organization. (1978). *Declaration of Alma-Ata.* Paper presented at the International Conference on Primary Health Care, Alma-Ata, USSR.

World Health Organization. (1979). *Global strategy for health for all by the year 2000: Based on the Alma-Ata report and Declaration in 1978.* Paper presented at the 32th World Health Assembly, Geneva.

World Health Organization. (1988). *Health promotion for working populations: Report of a World Health Organization expert committee* (Technical Report Series 765). Geneva: Author.

World Health Organization. (1998). *Health promotion glossary.* Geneva, Switzerland: World Health Organization.

World Health Organization. (1999). *Health 21: Health for all in the 21st century.* Copenhagen, Denmark: World Health Organization.

World Health Organization. (2001a). *Health promotion: Report by the Secretariat.* Fifty-fourth World Health Assembly, Geneva, Switzerland: World Health Organization.

World Health Organization. (2001b). *International classification of functioning, disability and health.* Geneva, Switzerland: World Health Organization.

World Health Organization. (2002, April). *Active aging: A policy framework.* Paper presented at the World Health Organization to the Second United Nations World Assembly on Aging, Madrid, Spain.

World Health Organization. (2003). *Diet, nutrition and the prevention of chronic diseases.* Geneva, Switzerland: World Health Organization.

Yamaki, K. (2005). Body weight status among adults with intellectual disability in the community. *Mental Retardation, 43*(1), 1–10.

Yamaki, K., & Fujiura, G.T. (2002). Employment and income status of adults with developmental disabilities living in the community. *Mental Retardation, 40*(2), 132–141.

YMCA of the USA. (2000). *YMCA fitness testing and assessment manual (4th ed).* Retrieved February 16, 2010, from http://www.exrx.net/Calculators/YBenchPress.html

Zarcadoolas, C., Pleasant, A., & Greer, D. (2006). *Advancing health literacy: A framework for understanding and action.* San Francisco: Jossey-Bass.

Health Matters Assessments

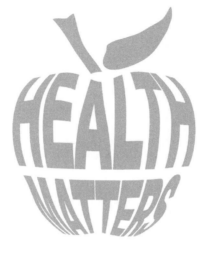

Sustaining Your Health Promotion Program

Contents

Health Matters Assessments, copyright © 2009 Beth Marks and Jasmina Sisirak, Rehabilitation Research
and Training Center on Aging with Developmental Disabilities, University of Illinois at Chicago.

In *Health Matters for People with Developmental Disabilities: Creating a Sustainable Health Promotion
Program*, by Beth Marks, Jasmina Sisirak, and Tamar Heller (2010, Paul H. Brookes Publishing Co.)

Introduction

The Health Matters Assessments (HMA) can be completed by employees of community-based day and residential organizations providing services for people with developmental disabilities (DD). The HMA packet will help you evaluate organizational **needs** and **capacity** for developing a health promotion plan including programs, services, environmental support, resources, culture, and employee knowledge and skills to do health-promoting activities.

How Will HMA Help You?

Evaluating your health promotion program can be beneficial in many ways:

1. Understand, verify, or increase the impact of services and programs for people with DD and staff. These "outcome" evaluations are increasingly required by nonprofit funders to verify that their monies are helping their constituents. Service providers can understand what their clients and employees need, evaluate their organizational capacity, and generate reports on how the new services could be delivered.

2. Benchmark your organization's capacity to promote health among your clients and employees. This will allow you to develop targeted, strategic action plans for health promotion programming.

3. Improve delivery mechanisms to be more efficient and less costly. Without program evaluation, service delivery may end up being an ineffective collection of activities that are less efficient and more costly than needed. Evaluations can identify program strengths and weaknesses to improve the program and to adapt and adjust it to meet the needs of people with DD and your organization.

4. Verify that you are doing what you think you are doing. Typically, plans about how to deliver programs and services end up changing substantially as those plans are put into place. Evaluations can verify if the program is really running as originally planned.

5. Facilitate what management is really thinking about what their program is all about, including its goals, how it meets it goals, and how it will know if it has met its goals or not.

6. Produce data or verify results that can be used to understand how your program helps participants, give feedback to participants and staff in the program, improve public relations, and promote your services in the community.

7. Generate valid comparisons between programs to decide which should be retained (e.g., in the face of pending budget cuts).

8. Fully examine and describe effective programs for replication elsewhere.

Health Matters
Assessment of Needs (HMAN)

Health Promotion Programs and Services

Available Programs and Services for Clients and Employees[1]

1. Does your organization offer employees any health promotion programs or services? (Circle yes or no.)

   a) Yes

   b) No

2. Indicate (circle yes or no) if the following health promotion programs or services are offered at your organization for staff and/or clients with developmental disabilities?

		If services are available, are they offered to	
		Clients with DD	**Staff**
a)	Healthy eating/nutrition classes	**Yes** **No**	Yes No	Yes No
b)	Individual nutrition or diet management counseling	**Yes** **No**	Yes No	Yes No
c)	Fitness assessments	**Yes** **No**	Yes No	Yes No
d)	Group exercise classes	**Yes** **No**	Yes No	Yes No
e)	Health risk screening (e.g., cholesterol, blood pressure, blood sugar, bone density)	**Yes** **No**	Yes No	Yes No
f)	Tobacco cessation classes	**Yes** **No**	Yes No	Yes No
g)	Team-building classes	**Yes** **No**	Yes No	Yes No
h)	Peer mentoring classes	**Yes** **No**	Yes No	Yes No
i)	Leadership skills classes	**Yes** **No**	Yes No	Yes No

[1]Marks, B., & Sisirak, J. (2008). *Available Programs and Services for Clients and Employees Scale.* University of Illinois at Chicago: Rehabilitation Research and Training Center on Aging with Developmental Disabilities.

Promotional Messages*[2] Please answer yes or no to the following questions about promotional messages for healthy behaviors or health promotion programs. Does your organization...(circle yes or no)

a)	Provide *healthy-eating-specific* messages to staff or clients, such as posters or brochures?	Yes	No
b)	Provide *physical activity or exercise messages* to staff or clients, such as posters or brochures?	Yes	No
c)	Promote the availability of onsite health promotion programs through at least two modes of communication? (e.g., newsletters, bulletin boards)?	Yes	No

Wellness Committee

1. Does your organization have a wellness committee? (Circle yes or no.)

   a) Yes

   b) No

Environmental Support for Health Promotion

Physical Environment for Physical Activity[3]

1. Does your organization assist with accessing facilities that enable staff and clients/residents to be physically active?

   a) Yes

   b) No

Are the following facilities (either at your organization or in the community) open to clients with DD and/or staff?		If these facilities are available, are they open to	
		Clients with DD	**Staff**
a) Locker room with showers	**Yes**	Yes	Yes
	No	No	No
b) Indoor area set aside specifically for exercise and physical activity	**Yes**	Yes	Yes
	No	No	No
c) Aerobic exercise equipment such as stationary cycles, or Stairmasters	**Yes**	Yes	Yes
	No	No	No
d) Strength training equipment	**Yes**	Yes	Yes
	No	No	No
e) Outdoor facilities such as a jogging trail	**Yes**	Yes	Yes
	No	No	No

[2]Marks, B., & Sisirak, J. (2008). *Promotional Messages.* University of Illinois at Chicago: Rehabilitation Research and Training Center on Aging with Developmental Disabilities.

[3]Marks, B., & Sisirak, J. (2008). *Physical Environment for Physical Activity.* University of Illinois at Chicago: Rehabilitation Research and Training Center on Aging with Developmental Disabilities.

Physical Environment for Healthy Food Choices[4]

1. Does your organization have a snack bar or food service for employees and clients/residents?

    a) Yes

    b) No

If yes, does the snack bar or food service usually have (on a daily basis):		If services available, are they offered to	
		Clients with DD	Staff
1) "Healthy" food alternatives?	**Yes**	Yes	Yes
	No	No	No
2) Fresh fruits or vegetables?	**Yes**	Yes	Yes
	No	No	No
3) "Healthy" beverage alternatives?	**Yes**	Yes	Yes
	No	No	No
4) Labels (e.g., "low-fat," "light," "heart healthy") to identify "healthy" food alternatives?	**Yes**	Yes	Yes
	No	No	No
5) Labels on foods indicating the basis of nutritional value (e.g., calories, fat grams, percent of calories from fat)?	**Yes**	Yes	Yes
	No	No	No

2. Does your organization have vending machines for employees and clients/residents to access food or beverages?

    a) Yes

    b) No

If yes, do the vending machines usually have:		If these items are in vending machines, are they available to:	
		Clients with DD	Staff
1) Fruits (dried or fresh), low fat snacks, or other "healthy" *food alternatives?*	**Yes**	Yes	Yes
	No	No	No
2) "Healthy" *beverage alternatives?*	**Yes**	Yes	Yes
	No	No	No

[4]Marks, B., & Sisirak, J. (2008). *Physical Environment for Healthy Food Choices*. University of Illinois at Chicago: Rehabilitation Research and Training Center on Aging with Developmental Disabilities.

Health Matters Assessments, copyright © 2009 Beth Marks and Jasmina Sisirak, Rehabilitation Research and Training Center on Aging with Developmental Disabilities, University of Illinois at Chicago.

In *Health Matters for People with Developmental Disabilities: Creating a Sustainable Health Promotion Program,* by Beth Marks, Jasmina Sisirak, and Tamar Heller (2010, Paul H. Brookes Publishing Co.)

If yes, do the vending machines usually have:		If these items are in vending machines, are they available to:	
		Clients with DD	Staff
3) Labels that identify *"healthy" foods alternatives* on or near the vending machines?	**Yes**	Yes	Yes
	No	No	No
4) Labels that indicate *nutritional value* provided on or near the vending machines (e.g., fat grams, percent of calories from fat)?	**Yes**	Yes	Yes
	No	No	No

Testing Procedure Manual

A needs assessment should simultaneously be done among potential participants with DD to prioritize health-related issues (e.g., overall health status, obesity rates, pain, depression, fitness levels, knowledge of exercise and health food choices, engaging in physical activity and making healthy food choices). Please refer to Appendix E in *Health Matters: The Exercise and Nutrition Health Education Curriculum for People with Developmental Disabilities* (Marks, Sisirak, & Heller, Paul H. Brookes Publishing Co., 2010).

Health Matters Assessment of Capacity (HMAC)

Resources

Organizational Resources Supporting Health Promotion[1]

1. Does your organization have resources to support your efforts in providing health promotion services (e.g., physical activity, eating more fruits and vegetables)?

Please circle how much you agree or disagree with the following statements:	Strongly disagree	Disagree	Agree	Strongly agree	Don't know
a) I have enough cooking-related equipment to prepare healthy meals with clients.	1	2	3	4	0
b) I have enough fitness-related supplies to do physical activities with clients.	1	2	3	4	0
c) I have support from my manager to do health promotion activities.	1	2	3	4	0
d) I have support from my coworkers to do health promotion activities.	1	2	3	4	0
e) I have access to financial resources that support health promotion activities for clients (e.g., gym memberships, adequate money to buy healthy food).	1	2	3	4	0
f) I have access to community resources that support health promotion activities for clients (e.g., parks, gyms, and healthy food sources and stores).	1	2	3	4	0
g) My workplace offers trainings on health promotion activities for people with I/DD.	1	2	3	4	0
h) My workplace offers trainings on health promotion activities for staff.	1	2	3	4	0

[1]Marks, B., & Sisirak, J. (2008). *Organizational Resources Supporting Health Promotion Scale.* University of Illinois at Chicago: Rehabilitation Research and Training Center on Aging with Developmental Disabilities.

Please circle how much you agree or disagree with the following statements:	Strongly disagree	Disagree	Agree	Strongly agree	Don't know
i) My workplace offers health promotion activities are available to people with DD.	1	2	3	4	0
j) My workplace offers health promotion activities and programs to staff.	1	2	3	4	0
k) My organization provides incentives for people with DD who participate in health promotion activities.	1	2	3	4	0
l) My organization provides incentives for staff who participate in employee health promotion programs.	1	2	3	4	0
m) My organization provides incentives for staff who support health promotion activities for people with DD.	1	2	3	4	0
n) My organization has funding (monies) to do health promotion activities.	1	2	3	4	0
o) My organization has adequate staffing to do health promotion activities.	1	2	3	4	0

Local Community Resources Supporting Health Promotion[2]

1. Does your organization have resources to support your efforts to provide health promotion services (e.g., physical activity, eating more fruits and vegetables)?

Please circle how much you agree or disagree with the following statements:	Strongly disagree	Disagree	Agree	Strongly agree	Don't know
a) We actively use community resources (e.g., recreation centers, universities, churches) to support our health promotion programs.	1	2	3	4	0

[2]Marks, B., & Sisirak, J. (2008). *Organizational Resources Supporting Health Promotion Scale.* Rehabilitation Research and Training Center on Aging with Developmental Disabilities, University of Illinois at Chicago.

Please circle how much you agree or disagree with the following statements:	Strongly disagree	Disagree	Agree	Strongly agree	Don't know
b) Community members (e.g., students, health professionals) volunteer at all levels of our organization to work in health promotion programs (e.g., run classes, board members).	1	2	3	4	0
c) We actively work with park districts and fitness centers in our community.	1	2	3	4	0

2. Does your organization provide a list of nearby restaurants with healthy food choices in their menus?

    a) Yes

    b) No

3. Does your organization provide a list of community-based activities and their associated fees?

    a) Yes

    b) No

Organizational Culture

1. Does your organization support your efforts to provide health promotion services (e.g., physical activity, more fruits and vegetables) through its commitment, policies, and structures?

Organizational Commitment[3]

Please circle how much you agree or disagree with the following statements:	Strongly disagree	Disagree	Agree	Strongly agree	Don't know
1) Health promotion is valued by everyone in our organization.	1	2	3	4	0
2) Our policies and programs support health promotion.	1	2	3	4	0

[3]Marks, B., & Sisirak, J. (2008). *Organizational Commitment Scale.* University of Illinois at Chicago: Rehabilitation Research and Training Center on Aging with Developmental Disabilities.

Please circle how much you agree or disagree with the following statements:	Strongly disagree	Disagree	Agree	Strongly agree	Don't know
3) We have strategic priorities related to health promotion.	1	2	3	4	0
4) We have partnerships with diverse organizations and communities supporting our health promotion programs (e.g., recreation centers, hospitals, universities).	1	2	3	4	0
5) Our leaders and managers support our health promotion programs.	1	2	3	4	0
6) Our staff support our health promotion programs.	1	2	3	4	0
7) Innovation and education in health promotion is strongly encouraged in our organization.	1	2	3	4	0
8) Employees collaborate to achieve health promotion goals.	1	2	3	4	0

Policies and Incentives[4]

Please circle how much you agree or disagree with the following statements:	Strongly disagree	Disagree	Agree	Strongly agree	Don't know
1) Our policies and programs support health promotion for people with DD.	1	2	3	4	0
2) Our policies and programs support our health promotion for staff.	1	2	3	4	0
3) Our leaders and managers are supportive in providing health promotion to people with DD.	1	2	3	4	0
4) We have clear communication about health promotion activities throughout our organization.	1	2	3	4	0
5) Health promotion responsibilities are clearly stated in job descriptions.	1	2	3	4	0

[4]Marks, B., & Sisirak, J. (2008). *Policies and Incentives Scale.* University of Illinois at Chicago: Rehabilitation Research and Training Center on Aging with Developmental Disabilities.

Please circle how much you agree or disagree with the following statements:	Strongly disagree	Disagree	Agree	Strongly agree	Don't know
6) Health promotion responsibilities are addressed in job performance reviews.	1	2	3	4	0
7) Health promotion activities are part of staff performance objectives.	1	2	3	4	0

Please answer the following questions about policies at your organization. Does your organization have policies that...	None	Informal	Written/ Formal	Don't know	Not applicable
1) Require healthy food preparation practices in the homes of people with DD (steaming, low fat/salt substitutes, limited frying)?					
2) Require healthy food options at the work site (snackbar, food service)					
3) Require healthy food options in the **vending machines**?					
4) Require healthy food options at **meetings and events**?					
5) Support staff physical activity (policies that allow workers additional time off from lunch to exercise, walk breaks)?					
6) Provide health promotion programs during work time?					
7) Discount memberships to off-site recreation or fitness facilities **for staff**?					
8) Reduce health insurance fees for staff who participate in healthy lifestyle activities?					
9) Include health promotion in your organization's vision and mission statement?					

Structures[5]

Please circle how much you agree or disagree with the following statements:	Strongly disagree	Disagree	Agree	Strongly agree	Don't know
1) Health promotion is a shared responsibility in the organization.	1	2	3	4	0
2) Designated person/department evaluates health promotion activities for **people with DD.**	1	2	3	4	0
3) Designated person/department evaluates health promotion activities **for staff.**	1	2	3	4	0
4) A handbook describing health promotion activities is available **for people with DD.**	1	2	3	4	0
5) A handbook describing health promotion activities is available **for staff.**	1	2	3	4	0

Perceived Workload[6]

Please circle how much you agree or disagree with the following statements:	Not at all	Just a little	Moderate amount	Quite a lot	A great deal
1) I do not have enough time to carry out my work.	1	2	3	4	5
2) I cannot meet all the conflicting demands made on my time at work.	1	2	3	4	5
3) I never finish work feeling that I have completed everything I should.	1	2	3	4	5
4) I am asked to do work without adequate resources to complete it.	1	2	3	4	5
5) I cannot follow best practice in the time available.	1	2	3	4	5
6) I am required to do basic tasks that prevent me from completing more important ones.	1	2	3	4	5

---

[5]Marks, B., & Sisirak, J. (2008). *Health Promotion Structures Scale.* University of Illinois at Chicago: Rehabilitation Research and Training Center on Aging with Developmental Disabilities.
[6]Caplan, R.D. (1971). *Organizational stress and individual strain: A social psychological study of risk factors in coronary heart disease among administrators, engineers, and scientists.* Ann Arbor: University of Michigan.

Employee Knowledge Related to Health Promotion[7]

What is your capacity to provide health promotion to adults with DD?

Please circle how much you agree or disagree with the following statements:	Strongly disagree	Disagree	Agree	Strongly agree	Don't know
1) I understand health risk factors related to persons with DD.	1	2	3	4	0
2) I think that health promotion is important for people with DD.	1	2	3	4	0
3) I use a variety of strategies to increase physical activity and healthy food choices for clients.	1	2	3	4	0
4) I may use different health promotion strategies depending on the needs of individual clients.	1	2	3	4	0
5) I consider personal preferences in **physical activities** for people with DD.	1	2	3	4	0
6) I consider personal preferences in **healthy food choices** for people with DD.	1	2	3	4	0
7) I believe that clients should participate in developing their personal health promotion goals.	1	2	3	4	0
8) I know **where to find** resources to learn more about physical activities.	1	2	3	4	0
9) I know **where to find** resources about nutrition.	1	2	3	4	0
10) I know **how to use** resources about physical activities.	1	2	3	4	0
11) I know **how to use** resources about nutrition.	1	2	3	4	0

[7]Marks, B., & Sisirak, J. (2008). *Employee Knowledge Related to Health Promotion Scale.* University of Illinois at Chicago: Rehabilitation Research and Training Center on Aging with Developmental Disabilities.

Employee Skills and Attitudes
Related to Health Promotion Activities

Do You Think You Can Do Health Promotion Activities?[8]

We would like to know how confident you are that you can do the following items:	Not at all confident				Totally confident
1) I am confident that I can **plan** a health promotion program (e.g., health education classes, exercise classes) for people with DD.	1	2	3	4	5
2) I am confident that I can **run** a health promotion program for people with DD.	1	2	3	4	5
3) I am confident that I can **evaluate** (e.g. improvements in health functions, behavior) a health promotion program for people with DD.	1	2	3	4	5
4) I am confident that I can **teach** people with DD how to do exercises to **increase their flexibility**.	1	2	3	4	5
5) I am confident that I can **teach** people with DD how to do exercises to **increase their strength and endurance** (e.g., using weight machines, few weights).	1	2	3	4	5
6) I am confident that I can **teach** people with DD how to do exercises to **increase their aerobic endurance** (e.g., walking, swimming, or bicycling).	1	2	3	4	5
7) I am confident that I can **teach** people with DD how to make **healthy food choices**.	1	2	3	4	5
8) I am confident that I can **teach** people with DD how to **eat more fruits and vegetables**.	1	2	3	4	5
9) I am confident that I can **teach** people with DD how to **choose healthy portion sizes**.	1	2	3	4	5
10) I am confident that I can **advocate** for health promotion.	1	2	3	4	5

---

[8]Marks, B., & Sisirak, J. (2008). *Self-Efficacy Related to Health Promotion Scale.* University of Illinois at Chicago: Rehabilitation Research and Training Center on Aging with Developmental Disabilities.

What Is Good About Exercising for People with DD?[9]

Please circle how much you agree or disagree that regular exercise would help people with DD to...	Strongly disagree	Disagree	Agree	Strongly agree
1) Lose or control their weight	1	2	3	4
2) Give them more energy	1	2	3	4
3) Make their bodies feel good physically	1	2	3	4
4) Make them feel good emotionally	1	2	3	4
5) Decrease their joint pain and stiffness	1	2	3	4
6) Meet new people	1	2	3	4
7) Get in shape	1	2	3	4
8) Look better	1	2	3	4
9) Improve their overall health	1	2	3	4
10) Reduce their cholesterol level	1	2	3	4
11) Reduce their blood pressure	1	2	3	4
12) Improve their endurance	1	2	3	4

Do You Think that People with DD Can Exercise?[10]

We want to know how confident you are that people with DD can...	Not at all confident				Totally confident
1) Do exercises to increase their flexibility	1	2	3	4	5
2) Do exercises to increase their strength and endurance (e.g., weight machines, free weights)	1	2	3	4	5
3) Do exercises to increase their aerobic endurance (e.g., walking, swimming, or bicycling)	1	2	3	4	5

---

[9]Heller, T., & Prochaska, T.J. (2001). *Exercise Perception Scale.* Rehabilitation Research and Training Center on Aging with Developmental Disabilities, University of Illinois at Chicago.

[10]Marks, B., & Sisirak, J. (2008). *Self-Efficacy Related to Exercise for People with DD Scale.* University of Illinois at Chicago: Rehabilitation Research and Training Center on Aging with Developmental Disabilities.

What Barriers Keep People with DD from Exercising?[11]

Please CIRCLE how much you agree or disagree that these barriers keep people with DD from exercising:	Strongly disagree	Disagree	Neither	Agree	Strongly agree
1) Costs too much money	1	2	3	4	5
2) Lack of transportation to an exercise program	1	2	3	4	5
3) Not enough time	1	2	3	4	5
4) Lack of interest	1	2	3	4	5
5) Lack of energy	1	2	3	4	5
6) Exercise is boring	1	2	3	4	5
7) Exercise will not improve their condition	1	2	3	4	5
8) Exercise will make their condition worse	1	2	3	4	5
9) Exercising is too difficult for them	1	2	3	4	5
10) They don't know how to exercise	1	2	3	4	5
11) They don't know where to exercise	1	2	3	4	5
12) Health concerns prevent them from exercising	1	2	3	4	5
13) They are too lazy to exercise	1	2	3	4	5
14) They don't have anyone to exercise with	1	2	3	4	5
15) The equipment is not made for someone with their disabilities	1	2	3	4	5
16) They worry that people might make fun of them	1	2	3	4	5
17) No one shows them how to exercise	1	2	3	4	5
18) Fitness centers are not accessible (i.e., they can't get in and around the center)	1	2	3	4	5

[11]Heller, T., Rimmer, J., & Rubin, S. (2001). *Barriers Scale.* University of Illinois at Chicago: Rehabilitation Research and Training Center on Aging with Developmental Disabilities.

What's Good About Eating Fruits and Vegetables for People with DD?[12]

Please circle how much you agree or disagree that if people with DD eat *fruits* and *vegetables every day* it would...

		I disagree very much	I disagree a little	I'm not sure	I agree a little	I agree very much
1)	Help them lose or control weight	1	2	3	4	5
2)	Give them more energy	1	2	3	4	5
3)	Reduce constipation	1	2	3	4	5
4)	Make them feel stronger	1	2	3	4	5
5)	Improve their overall health	1	2	3	4	5
6)	Improve their cholesterol level	1	2	3	4	5
7)	Improve their blood pressure	1	2	3	4	5

Do You Think that People with DD Can Make Healthy Food Choices?[13]

We would like to know how confident you are that people with DD can do the following at home or work...

		Not at all confident				Totally confident
1)	Eat more fruits and vegetables	1	2	3	4	5
2)	Eat at least 5–9 servings of fruits and vegetables each day	1	2	3	4	5
3)	Make healthy food choices	1	2	3	4	5
4)	Eat favorite fruit instead of usual dessert	1	2	3	4	5
5)	Choose healthy portion sizes	1	2	3	4	5

---

[12]Sisirak, J., & Marks, B. (2008). *Fruit and Vegetable Outcome Expectations Scale.* University of Illinois at Chicago: Rehabilitation Research and Training Center on Aging with Developmental Disabilities.

[13]Sisirak, J., & Marks, B. (2008). *Fruit and Vegetable Self-Efficacy Scale.* University of Illinois at Chicago: Rehabilitation Research and Training Center on Aging with Developmental Disabilities.

What Keeps People with DD from Eating Fruits and Vegetables?[14]

We would like to know what keeps people with DD from eating fruits and vegetables. Please circle how much you agree or disagree that the following *barriers keep* people with DD from *eating fruits and vegetables*:

		Strongly disagree	Disagree	Agree	Strongly agree
1)	Cost too much money	1	2	3	4
2)	Take too much time to prepare	1	2	3	4
3)	Will not improve their health	1	2	3	4
4)	Will make their health worse	1	2	3	4
5)	Are too difficult to chew and swallow	1	2	3	4
6)	Are too hard to prepare	1	2	3	4
7)	Are hard to buy because they don't know how	1	2	3	4
8)	Are hard to prepare because they are too lazy	1	2	3	4
9)	Are hard to prepare because there's no one to show them how to prepare them	1	2	3	4
10)	Go bad too quickly	1	2	3	4
11)	Are hard to buy because they don't know what is in season	1	2	3	4
12)	Do not have as much nutritional value as canned fruit and vegetables	1	2	3	4
13)	Do not taste as good as canned fruit and vegetables	1	2	3	4
14)	Do not taste good to them	1	2	3	4
15)	Will not be eaten by their family	1	2	3	4

---

[14]Sisirak, J., & Marks, B. (2008). *Barriers to Eating Fruits and Vegetables Scale.* University of Illinois at Chicago: Rehabilitation Research and Training Center on Aging with Developmental Disabilities.

Demographics

1. **What is your current position?**
   a. Case worker
   b. Dietary
   c. Direct support professional (DSP)
   d. Housekeeping
   e. Instructor
   f. Job coach
   g. Management
   h. Nurse
   i. Office support staff
   j. QMRP
   k. Residential teacher
   l. Security
   m. Social worker
   n. Supervisor
   o. Therapist (OT, PT)
   p. Other

2. **Where do you work?**
   a) Residential
   b) Supported living
   c) Assisted living
   d) Day activity
   e) Supported employment
   f) Other_____

3. **How many clients does your organization serve annually?**
   a) Less than 100
   b) 100–500
   c) Greater than 500

4. **Does your organization provide residential services, day services, or both?**
   a) Residential services only
   b) Day services only
   c) Both residential services and day services

5. **What is your annual turnover rate?**
   a) < 25 %
   b) 25%–50%
   c) 51%–75%
   d) > 75%

6. **Your age:** _____ years

7. **What is your gender?**

   1 Female   2 Male

8. **What is the highest grade of school that you completed? (Please circle one response.)**

   1 Less than 8th grade
   2 8th-grade graduate
   3 Some high school (Grades 9–12)
   4 High school graduate
   5 Some college
   6 College graduate
   7 Post-college or graduate school

9. **What race/ethnicity do you consider yourself? (Please circle only one response)**

   1 American Indian or Alaskan Native
   2 Asian or Pacific Islander
   3 Black, not of Hispanic origin
   4 Hispanic/Latino
   5 White, not of Hispanic origin
   6 Other (Please specify)
   _____

10. **How long have you worked in this organization?**

    _____Years _____ Months

11. **How long have you worked with people with DD?**

    _____ Years _____ Month

Index

Page numbers followed by *f* indicate figures; those followed by *t* indicate tables.